GIANT CELL ARTERITIS

A MEDICAL DICTIONARY, BIBLIOGRAPHY,
AND ANNOTATED RESEARCH GUIDE TO
INTERNET REFERENCES

JAMES N. PARKER, M.D.
AND PHILIP M. PARKER, PH.D., EDITORS

ii

ICON Health Publications
ICON Group International, Inc.
4370 La Jolla Village Drive, 4th Floor
San Diego, CA 92122 USA

Printed in the United States of America.

Last digit indicates print number: 10 9 8 7 6 4 5 3 2 1

Publisher, Health Care: Philip Parker, Ph.D.
Editor(s): James Parker, M.D., Philip Parker, Ph.D.

Publisher's note: The ideas, procedures, and suggestions contained in this book are not intended for the diagnosis or treatment of a health problem. As new medical or scientific information becomes available from academic and clinical research, recommended treatments and drug therapies may undergo changes. The authors, editors, and publisher have attempted to make the information in this book up to date and accurate in accord with accepted standards at the time of publication. The authors, editors, and publisher are not responsible for errors or omissions or for consequences from application of the book, and make no warranty, expressed or implied, in regard to the contents of this book. Any practice described in this book should be applied by the reader in accordance with professional standards of care used in regard to the unique circumstances that may apply in each situation. The reader is advised to always check product information (package inserts) for changes and new information regarding dosage and contraindications before prescribing any drug or pharmacological product. Caution is especially urged when using new or infrequently ordered drugs, herbal remedies, vitamins and supplements, alternative therapies, complementary therapies and medicines, and integrative medical treatments.

Cataloging-in-Publication Data

Parker, James N., 1961-
Parker, Philip M., 1960-

Giant Cell Arteritis: A Medical Dictionary, Bibliography, and Annotated Research Guide to Internet References / James N. Parker and Philip M. Parker, editors
        p.   cm.
Includes bibliographical references, glossary, and index.
ISBN: 0-497-00476-3
1. Giant Cell Arteritis-Popular works. I. Title.

Disclaimer

This publication is not intended to be used for the diagnosis or treatment of a health problem. It is sold with the understanding that the publisher, editors, and authors are not engaging in the rendering of medical, psychological, financial, legal, or other professional services.

References to any entity, product, service, or source of information that may be contained in this publication should not be considered an endorsement, either direct or implied, by the publisher, editors, or authors. ICON Group International, Inc., the editors, and the authors are not responsible for the content of any Web pages or publications referenced in this publication.

Copyright Notice

Acknowledgements

The collective knowledge generated from academic and applied research summarized in various references has been critical in the creation of this book which is best viewed as a comprehensive compilation and collection of information prepared by various official agencies which produce publications on giant cell arteritis. Books in this series draw from various agencies and institutions associated with the United States Department of Health and Human Services, and in particular, the Office of the Secretary of Health and Human Services (OS), the Administration for Children and Families (ACF), the Administration on Aging (AOA), the Agency for Healthcare Research and Quality (AHRQ), the Agency for Toxic Substances and Disease Registry (ATSDR), the Centers for Disease Control and Prevention (CDC), the Food and Drug Administration (FDA), the Healthcare Financing Administration (HCFA), the Health Resources and Services Administration (HRSA), the Indian Health Service (IHS), the institutions of the National Institutes of Health (NIH), the Program Support Center (PSC), and the Substance Abuse and Mental Health Services Administration (SAMHSA). In addition to these sources, information gathered from the National Library of Medicine, the United States Patent Office, the European Union, and their related organizations has been invaluable in the creation of this book. Some of the work represented was financially supported by the Research and Development Committee at INSEAD. This support is gratefully acknowledged. Finally, special thanks are owed to Tiffany Freeman for her excellent editorial support.

About the Editors

James N. Parker, M.D.

Dr. James N. Parker received his Bachelor of Science degree in Psychobiology from the University of California, Riverside and his M.D. from the University of California, San Diego. In addition to authoring numerous research publications, he has lectured at various academic institutions. Dr. Parker is the medical editor for health books by ICON Health Publications.

Philip M. Parker, Ph.D.

Philip M. Parker is the Eli Lilly Chair Professor of Innovation, Business and Society at INSEAD (Fontainebleau, France and Singapore). Dr. Parker has also been Professor at the University of California, San Diego and has taught courses at Harvard University, the Hong Kong University of Science and Technology, the Massachusetts Institute of Technology, Stanford University, and UCLA. Dr. Parker is the associate editor for ICON Health Publications.

About ICON Health Publications

To discover more about ICON Health Publications, simply check with your preferred online booksellers, including Barnes&Noble.com and Amazon.com which currently carry all of our titles. Or, feel free to contact us directly for bulk purchases or institutional discounts:

ICON Group International, Inc.
4370 La Jolla Village Drive, Fourth Floor
San Diego, CA 92122 USA
Fax: 858-546-4341
Web site: **www.icongrouponline.com/health**

Table of Contents

FORWARD

In March 2001, the National Institutes of Health issued the following warning: "The number of Web sites offering health-related resources grows every day. Many sites provide valuable information, while others may have information that is unreliable or misleading."[1] Furthermore, because of the rapid increase in Internet-based information, many hours can be wasted searching, selecting, and printing. Since only the smallest fraction of information dealing with giant cell arteritis is indexed in search engines, such as **www.google.com** or others, a non-systematic approach to Internet research can be not only time consuming, but also incomplete. This book was created for medical professionals, students, and members of the general public who want to know as much as possible about giant cell arteritis, using the most advanced research tools available and spending the least amount of time doing so.

In addition to offering a structured and comprehensive bibliography, the pages that follow will tell you where and how to find reliable information covering virtually all topics related to giant cell arteritis, from the essentials to the most advanced areas of research. Public, academic, government, and peer-reviewed research studies are emphasized. Various abstracts are reproduced to give you some of the latest official information available to date on giant cell arteritis. Abundant guidance is given on how to obtain free-of-charge primary research results via the Internet. **While this book focuses on the field of medicine, when some sources provide access to non-medical information relating to giant cell arteritis, these are noted in the text.**

E-book and electronic versions of this book are fully interactive with each of the Internet sites mentioned (clicking on a hyperlink automatically opens your browser to the site indicated). If you are using the hard copy version of this book, you can access a cited Web site by typing the provided Web address directly into your Internet browser. You may find it useful to refer to synonyms or related terms when accessing these Internet databases. **NOTE:** At the time of publication, the Web addresses were functional. However, some links may fail due to URL address changes, which is a common occurrence on the Internet.

For readers unfamiliar with the Internet, detailed instructions are offered on how to access electronic resources. For readers unfamiliar with medical terminology, a comprehensive glossary is provided. For readers without access to Internet resources, a directory of medical libraries, that have or can locate references cited here, is given. We hope these resources will prove useful to the widest possible audience seeking information on giant cell arteritis.

The Editors

---

[1] From the NIH, National Cancer Institute (NCI): **http://www.cancer.gov/cancerinfo/ten-things-to-know**.

CHAPTER 1. STUDIES ON GIANT CELL ARTERITIS

Overview

In this chapter, we will show you how to locate peer-reviewed references and studies on giant cell arteritis.

The Combined Health Information Database

The Combined Health Information Database summarizes studies across numerous federal agencies. To limit your investigation to research studies and giant cell arteritis, you will need to use the advanced search options. First, go to **http://chid.nih.gov/index.html**. From there, select the "Detailed Search" option (or go directly to that page with the following hyperlink: **http://chid.nih.gov/detail/detail.html**). The trick in extracting studies is found in the drop boxes at the bottom of the search page where "You may refine your search by." Select the dates and language you prefer, and the format option "Journal Article." At the top of the search form, select the number of records you would like to see (we recommend 100) and check the box to display "whole records." We recommend that you type "giant cell arteritis" (or synonyms) into the "For these words:" box. Consider using the option "anywhere in record" to make your search as broad as possible. If you want to limit the search to only a particular field, such as the title of the journal, then select this option in the "Search in these fields" drop box. The following is what you can expect from this type of search:

- **Jaw Claudication: A Sign of Giant Cell Arteritis**

  Source: JADA. Journal of American Dental Association. 126(7): 1028-1029. July 1995.

  Summary: Giant cell arteritis (GCA) is a polysymptomatic disease with manifestations that include headaches, joint pains, scalp tenderness, fever, malaise, and weight loss. This article presents a case report that describes a patient with jaw claudication as the initial sign of **giant cell arteritis.** Visual loss, usually due to ischemic optic neuropathy, is the major complication of this disorder, and early diagnosis and treatment are critical. The author stresses that dentists should consider jaw claudication when making the differential diagnosis of jaw pain, especially in the elderly patient. 5 references. (AA-M).

Federally Funded Research on Giant Cell Arteritis

The U.S. Government supports a variety of research studies relating to giant cell arteritis. These studies are tracked by the Office of Extramural Research at the National Institutes of Health.[2] CRISP (Computerized Retrieval of Information on Scientific Projects) is a searchable database of federally funded biomedical research projects conducted at universities, hospitals, and other institutions.

Search the CRISP Web site at **http://crisp.cit.nih.gov/crisp/crisp_query.generate_screen**. You will have the option to perform targeted searches by various criteria, including geography, date, and topics related to giant cell arteritis.

For most of the studies, the agencies reporting into CRISP provide summaries or abstracts. As opposed to clinical trial research using patients, many federally funded studies use animals or simulated models to explore giant cell arteritis. The following is typical of the type of information found when searching the CRISP database for giant cell arteritis:

- **Project Title: OCULAR DISEASE IN GIANT CELL ARTERITIS**

    Principal Investigator & Institution: Weyand, Cornelia M.; Director; Mayo Clinic Coll of Medicine, Rochester 200 1St St Sw Rochester, Mn 55905

    Timing: Fiscal Year 2002; Project Start 01-AUG-1997; Project End 31-JUL-2006

    Summary: (provided by applicant): **Giant cell arteritis** (GCA) is a sight-threatening systemic vasculitis with an immune-mediated pathogenesis. Vascular lesions, composed of activated T cells and macrophages, induce progressive, insidious vascular occlusion of medium-size arteries, resulting in tissue ischemia, such as ischemic optic neuropathy. Our long-term objective has been to unravel the mechanisms by which lymphocytes and macrophages are recruited to the vessel wall, differentiate into specialized effector cells, and promote GCA. During the last four years, we have made progress towards these goals by dissecting macrophage effector pathways that lead to arterial injury and the artery's response-to-injury program. Most importantly, we have provided evidence that the primary defect in GCA is a breach of T-cell tolerance and that T-cell activation occurs in the adventitia where dendritic cells (DC) initiate and maintain T-cell stimulation. We hypothesize that adventitial DC are key players in generating immunological privilege for the artery and that breakdown of this immune protection causes GCA. This hypothesis includes that structural and cellular components of the adventitia create the unique target-tissue susceptibility and age-dependence of GCA. Experiments to test this hypothesis will use a temporal artery-NOD/LtSz-Rag1 (tm1 Mom) mouse chimera model. The specific aims of this proposal are to: 1) Examine the heterogeneity of adventitial DC and vasa vasorum networks in different vascular beds and at different ages. Three-dimensional rendering of capillary networks in the adventitia and their relationship to DC indigenous to the adventitia will be examined by microcomputed-CT to define a model for the targeting of GCA to extracranial arteries in elderly individuals. 2) Determine the mechanisms of immune tolerance promoted by adventitial DC. These experiments will use adoptively transferred T cells in mouse chimeras. 3) Investigate the functional profile of adventitial DC in GCA and polymyalgia rheumatica (PMR), a forme fruste of GCA. Disease-relevant defects in DC function will be identified by gene

---

[2] Healthcare projects are funded by the National Institutes of Health (NIH), Substance Abuse and Mental Health Services (SAMHSA), Health Resources and Services Administration (HRSA), Food and Drug Administration (FDA), Centers for Disease Control and Prevention (CDCP), Agency for Healthcare Research and Quality (AHRQ), and Office of Assistant Secretary of Health (OASH).

expression profiling. 4) Explore the mechanisms of inappropriate arrest and premature differentiation of DC in PMR and GCA arteries. These studies will focus on pathways regulating the life cycle of DC and deviations leading to vasculitis. 5) Explore the therapeutic implications of modulating DC function in GCA. We will proceed with two approaches, TNF-alpha inhibitors and tolerogenic DC, in the attempt to disrupt persistent DC and T-cell activation in GCA. These experiments will help us understand the immunobiology of healthy and inflamed arteries, advance our understanding of the events initiating vasculitis, and may provide new avenues for therapeutic intervention.

Website: http://crisp.cit.nih.gov/crisp/Crisp_Query.Generate_Screen

- **Project Title: PULSE IV GLUCOCORTICOID INFUSION AS INITIAL TREATMENT OF GIANT CELL ARTERITIS**

Principal Investigator & Institution: Mazlumzadeh, Mehrdad; Mayo Clinic Coll of Medicine, Rochester 200 1St St Sw Rochester, Mn 55905

Timing: Fiscal Year 2002

Summary: Giant Cell Arteritis (GCA, temporal arteritis) is a vasculitis of the medium and large-sized arteries that usually presents with headache and visual disturbances in patients over the age of fifty. Conventional treatment with oral glucocorticoid (GC, steroid, prednisone) for up to two to three years has been the only known efficacious therapy to suppress the inflammatory process and prevent associated vascular complications. However, the long duration and the cumulative dose of GC therapy frequently results in multiple adverse effect. Recent studies have shown several relapses and persistence of inflammation based on elevated inflammatory markers such as interleulin-6 despite timely oral GC therapy. Investigations on animal models suggest the need for much higher doses of GC to appropriately treat the vasculitic process. This forms the basis of our proposed study which is a randomized, double-blinded, placebo-controlled, prospective clinical trial where biopsy proven GCA patients will be treated with high dose pulse intravenous (IV) GC initially followed by lower doses of oral GC. We hypothesize that this will result in shorter length of therapy with lower dose of GC and hence reduced adverse effects.

Website: http://crisp.cit.nih.gov/crisp/Crisp_Query.Generate_Screen

E-Journals: PubMed Central[3]

PubMed Central (PMC) is a digital archive of life sciences journal literature developed and managed by the National Center for Biotechnology Information (NCBI) at the U.S. National Library of Medicine (NLM).[4] Access to this growing archive of e-journals is free and unrestricted.[5] To search, go to **http://www.ncbi.nlm.nih.gov/entrez/query.fcgi?db=Pmc**, and type "giant cell arteritis" (or synonyms) into the search box. This search gives you access to full-text articles. The following is a sample of items found for giant cell arteritis in the PubMed Central database:

---

[3] Adapted from the National Library of Medicine: **http://www.pubmedcentral.nih.gov/about/intro.html**.

[4] With PubMed Central, NCBI is taking the lead in preservation and maintenance of open access to electronic literature, just as NLM has done for decades with printed biomedical literature. PubMed Central aims to become a world-class library of the digital age.

[5] The value of PubMed Central, in addition to its role as an archive, lies in the availability of data from diverse sources stored in a common format in a single repository. Many journals already have online publishing operations, and there is a growing tendency to publish material online only, to the exclusion of print.

- **Genetic epidemiology: Giant cell arteritis and polymyalgia rheumatica.** by Gonzalez-Gay MA.; 2001;
  http://www.pubmedcentral.gov/articlerender.fcgi?tool=pmcentrez&artid=128892

The National Library of Medicine: PubMed

One of the quickest and most comprehensive ways to find academic studies in both English and other languages is to use PubMed, maintained by the National Library of Medicine.[6] The advantage of PubMed over previously mentioned sources is that it covers a greater number of domestic and foreign references. It is also free to use. If the publisher has a Web site that offers full text of its journals, PubMed will provide links to that site, as well as to sites offering other related data. User registration, a subscription fee, or some other type of fee may be required to access the full text of articles in some journals.

To generate your own bibliography of studies dealing with giant cell arteritis, simply go to the PubMed Web site at **http://www.ncbi.nlm.nih.gov/pubmed**. Type "giant cell arteritis" (or synonyms) into the search box, and click "Go." The following is the type of output you can expect from PubMed for giant cell arteritis (hyperlinks lead to article summaries):

- **A multicenter, randomized, double-blind, placebo-controlled trial of adjuvant methotrexate treatment for giant cell arteritis.**
  Author(s): Hoffman GS, Cid MC, Hellmann DB, Guillevin L, Stone JH, Schousboe J, Cohen P, Calabrese LH, Dickler H, Merkel PA, Fortin P, Flynn JA, Locker GA, Easley KA, Schned E, Hunder GG, Sneller MC, Tuggle C, Swanson H, Hernandez-Rodriguez J, Lopez-Soto A, Bork D, Hoffman DB, Kalunian K, Klashman D, Wilke WS, Scheetz RJ, Mandell BF, Fessler BJ, Kosmorsky G, Prayson R, Luqmani RA, Nuki G, McRorie E, Sherrer Y, Baca S, Walsh B, Ferland D, Soubrier M, Choi HK, Gross W, Segal AM, Ludivico C, Puechal X; International Network for the Study of Systemic Vasculitides.
  Source: Arthritis and Rheumatism. 2002 May; 46(5): 1309-18.
  http://www.ncbi.nlm.nih.gov/entrez/query.fcgi?cmd=Retrieve&db=pubmed&dopt=Abstract&list_uids=12115238

- **A new medical diagnosis of Adolf Hitler. Giant cell arteritis-temporal arteritis.**
  Author(s): Redlich FC.
  Source: Archives of Internal Medicine. 1993 March 22; 153(6): 693-7.
  http://www.ncbi.nlm.nih.gov/entrez/query.fcgi?cmd=Retrieve&db=pubmed&dopt=Abstract&list_uids=8447705

- **A prospective, double-blind, randomized, placebo controlled trial of methotrexate in the treatment of giant cell arteritis (GCA).**
  Author(s): Spiera RF, Mitnick HJ, Kupersmith M, Richmond M, Spiera H, Peterson MG, Paget SA.
  Source: Clin Exp Rheumatol. 2001 September-October; 19(5): 495-501.
  http://www.ncbi.nlm.nih.gov/entrez/query.fcgi?cmd=Retrieve&db=pubmed&dopt=Abstract&list_uids=11579707

---

[6] PubMed was developed by the National Center for Biotechnology Information (NCBI) at the National Library of Medicine (NLM) at the National Institutes of Health (NIH). The PubMed database was developed in conjunction with publishers of biomedical literature as a search tool for accessing literature citations and linking to full-text journal articles at Web sites of participating publishers. Publishers that participate in PubMed supply NLM with their citations electronically prior to or at the time of publication.

- A randomized, multicenter, controlled trial using intravenous pulses of methylprednisolone in the initial treatment of simple forms of giant cell arteritis: a one year followup study of 164 patients.
  Author(s): Chevalet P, Barrier JH, Pottier P, Magadur-Joly G, Pottier MA, Hamidou M, Planchon B, El Kouri D, Connan L, Dupond JL, De Wazieres B, Dien G, Duhamel E, Grosbois B, Jego P, Le Strat A, Capdeville J, Letellier P, Agron L.
  Source: The Journal of Rheumatology. 2000 June; 27(6): 1484-91.
  http://www.ncbi.nlm.nih.gov/entrez/query.fcgi?cmd=Retrieve&db=pubmed&dopt=Abstract&list_uids=10852275

- Absence of detection of varicella-zoster virus DNA in temporal artery biopsies obtained from patients with giant cell arteritis.
  Author(s): Kennedy PG, Grinfeld E, Esiri MM.
  Source: Journal of the Neurological Sciences. 2003 November 15; 215(1-2): 27-9.
  http://www.ncbi.nlm.nih.gov/entrez/query.fcgi?cmd=Retrieve&db=pubmed&dopt=Abstract&list_uids=14568124

- Actinic granuloma in association with giant cell arteritis: are both caused by sunlight?
  Author(s): Lau H, Reid BJ, Weedon D.
  Source: Pathology. 1997 August; 29(3): 260-2.
  http://www.ncbi.nlm.nih.gov/entrez/query.fcgi?cmd=Retrieve&db=pubmed&dopt=Abstract&list_uids=9271011

- Acute angle-closure glaucoma in giant cell arteritis.
  Author(s): Kranemann CF, Buys YM.
  Source: Can J Ophthalmol. 1997 October; 32(6): 389-91. No Abstract Available.
  http://www.ncbi.nlm.nih.gov/entrez/query.fcgi?cmd=Retrieve&db=pubmed&dopt=Abstract&list_uids=9363343

- An unusual case of giant cell arteritis.
  Author(s): Shah P, Murray PI, Harry J.
  Source: American Journal of Ophthalmology. 1993 March 15; 115(3): 393-4.
  http://www.ncbi.nlm.nih.gov/entrez/query.fcgi?cmd=Retrieve&db=pubmed&dopt=Abstract&list_uids=8442503

- Analysis of the B cell repertoire against autoantigens in patients with giant cell arteritis and polymyalgia rheumatica.
  Author(s): Schmits R, Kubuschok B, Schuster S, Preuss KD, Pfreundschuh M.
  Source: Clinical and Experimental Immunology. 2002 February; 127(2): 379-85.
  http://www.ncbi.nlm.nih.gov/entrez/query.fcgi?cmd=Retrieve&db=pubmed&dopt=Abstract&list_uids=11876765

- ANCA-associated giant cell arteritis presenting with mononeuritis multiplex and central retinal artery occlusion: a case report.
  Author(s): Chan WM, Liu DT, Chan AY, Lai CH, Choi PC, Lam DS.
  Source: Rheumatology (Oxford, England). 2004 April; 43(4): 529-31.
  http://www.ncbi.nlm.nih.gov/entrez/query.fcgi?cmd=Retrieve&db=pubmed&dopt=Abstract&list_uids=15024142

- **Antiphospholipid antibodies and thrombophilic factors in giant cell arteritis.**
  Author(s): Espinosa G, Tassies D, Font J, Munoz-Rodriguez FJ, Cervera R, Ordinas A, Reverter JC, Ingelmo M.
  Source: Seminars in Arthritis and Rheumatism. 2001 August; 31(1): 12-20.
  http://www.ncbi.nlm.nih.gov/entrez/query.fcgi?cmd=Retrieve&db=pubmed&dopt=Abstract&list_uids=11503135

- **Anti-tumour necrosis factor treatment with infliximab in a case of giant cell arteritis resistant to steroid and immunosuppressive drugs.**
  Author(s): Airo P, Antonioli CM, Vianelli M, Toniati P.
  Source: Rheumatology (Oxford, England). 2002 March; 41(3): 347-9.
  http://www.ncbi.nlm.nih.gov/entrez/query.fcgi?cmd=Retrieve&db=pubmed&dopt=Abstract&list_uids=11934977

- **Aortic aneurysm and dissection are not associated with an increased risk for giant cell arteritis/ polymyalgia rheumatica.**
  Author(s): Ehrenfeld M, Bitzur R, Schneiderman J, Smolinsky A, Sidi Y, Gur H.
  Source: Postgraduate Medical Journal. 2000 July; 76(897): 409-11.
  http://www.ncbi.nlm.nih.gov/entrez/query.fcgi?cmd=Retrieve&db=pubmed&dopt=Abstract&list_uids=10878198

- **Aortic root replacement with a stentless bioprosthesis in a patient with giant cell arteritis.**
  Author(s): Iguchi A, Nitta Y, Saito T, Tabayashi K.
  Source: Jpn J Thorac Cardiovasc Surg. 2003 September; 51(9): 472-4.
  http://www.ncbi.nlm.nih.gov/entrez/query.fcgi?cmd=Retrieve&db=pubmed&dopt=Abstract&list_uids=14529171

- **Arterial wall production of cytokines in giant cell arteritis: results of a pilot study using human temporal artery cultures.**
  Author(s): Blain H, Abdelmouttaleb I, Belmin J, Blain A, Floquet J, Gueant JL, Jeandel C.
  Source: The Journals of Gerontology. Series A, Biological Sciences and Medical Sciences. 2002 April; 57(4): M241-5.
  http://www.ncbi.nlm.nih.gov/entrez/query.fcgi?cmd=Retrieve&db=pubmed&dopt=Abstract&list_uids=11909890

- **Association between infection and onset of giant cell arteritis: can seasonal patterns provide the answer?**
  Author(s): Liozon E, Loustaud V, Ly K, Vidal E.
  Source: The Journal of Rheumatology. 2001 May; 28(5): 1197-8.
  http://www.ncbi.nlm.nih.gov/entrez/query.fcgi?cmd=Retrieve&db=pubmed&dopt=Abstract&list_uids=11361213

- **Association of giant cell arteritis and polymyalgia rheumatica with different tumor necrosis factor microsatellite polymorphisms.**
  Author(s): Mattey DL, Hajeer AH, Dababneh A, Thomson W, Gonzalez-Gay MA, Garcia-Porrua C, Ollier WE.
  Source: Arthritis and Rheumatism. 2000 August; 43(8): 1749-55.
  http://www.ncbi.nlm.nih.gov/entrez/query.fcgi?cmd=Retrieve&db=pubmed&dopt=Abstract&list_uids=10943865

- **Atypical giant cell arteritis resulting in arm amputation.**
  Author(s): Cohen HE, Shankar PJ, Martin JC, Lewis MH.
  Source: Annals of the Royal College of Surgeons of England. 2003 July; 85(4): 260-2.
  http://www.ncbi.nlm.nih.gov/entrez/query.fcgi?cmd=Retrieve&db=pubmed&dopt=Abstract&list_uids=12855030

- **Audiovestibular manifestations in giant cell arteritis: a prospective study.**
  Author(s): Amor-Dorado JC, Llorca J, Garcia-Porrua C, Costa C, Perez-Fernandez N, Gonzalez-Gay MA.
  Source: Medicine; Analytical Reviews of General Medicine, Neurology, Psychiatry, Dermatology, and Pediatrics. 2003 January; 82(1): 13-26.
  http://www.ncbi.nlm.nih.gov/entrez/query.fcgi?cmd=Retrieve&db=pubmed&dopt=Abstract&list_uids=12544707

- **Audit of the management of suspected giant cell arteritis in a large teaching hospital.**
  Author(s): Dalbeth N, Lynch N, McLean L, McQueen F, Zwi J.
  Source: Internal Medicine Journal. 2002 July; 32(7): 315-9.
  http://www.ncbi.nlm.nih.gov/entrez/query.fcgi?cmd=Retrieve&db=pubmed&dopt=Abstract&list_uids=12088349

- **Basal and stimulated elastolytic activity of blood monocytes is increased in glucocorticoid-treated giant cell arteritis.**
  Author(s): Jensen HS, Mogensen HH, Mikkelsen AG.
  Source: Scandinavian Journal of Rheumatology. 1990; 19(4): 251-6.
  http://www.ncbi.nlm.nih.gov/entrez/query.fcgi?cmd=Retrieve&db=pubmed&dopt=Abstract&list_uids=2402598

- **Benefit or risk of aspirin treatment of giant cell arteritis: comment on the article by Weyand et al.**
  Author(s): Rothschild BM.
  Source: Arthritis and Rheumatism. 2002 November; 46(11): 3113; Author Reply 3113-4.
  http://www.ncbi.nlm.nih.gov/entrez/query.fcgi?cmd=Retrieve&db=pubmed&dopt=Abstract&list_uids=12428270

- **Bilateral internuclear ophthalmoplegia: an initial presenting sign of giant cell arteritis.**
  Author(s): Ahmad I, Zaman M.
  Source: Journal of the American Geriatrics Society. 1999 June; 47(6): 734-6. Review.
  http://www.ncbi.nlm.nih.gov/entrez/query.fcgi?cmd=Retrieve&db=pubmed&dopt=Abstract&list_uids=10366177

- **Bilateral internuclear ophthalmoplegia--an unusual initial presenting sign of giant cell arteritis.**
  Author(s): Crompton JL, Burrow DJ, Iyer PV.
  Source: Australian and New Zealand Journal of Ophthalmology. 1989 February; 17(1): 71-4.
  http://www.ncbi.nlm.nih.gov/entrez/query.fcgi?cmd=Retrieve&db=pubmed&dopt=Abstract&list_uids=2765284

- **Bilateral lower limb gangrene and stroke as initial manifestations of systemic giant cell arteritis in an African-American.**
  Author(s): Lie JT, Tokugawa DA.
  Source: The Journal of Rheumatology. 1995 February; 22(2): 363-6.
  http://www.ncbi.nlm.nih.gov/entrez/query.fcgi?cmd=Retrieve&db=pubmed&dopt=Abstract&list_uids=7738967

- **Bilateral ocular ischemic syndrome secondary to giant cell arteritis progressing despite corticosteroid treatment.**
  Author(s): Hwang JM, Girkin CA, Perry JD, Lai JC, Miller NR, Hellmann DB.
  Source: American Journal of Ophthalmology. 1999 January; 127(1): 102-4.
  http://www.ncbi.nlm.nih.gov/entrez/query.fcgi?cmd=Retrieve&db=pubmed&dopt=Abstract&list_uids=9933015

- **Bilateral ocular ischemic syndrome secondary to giant cell arteritis.**
  Author(s): Casson RJ, Fleming FK, Shaikh A, James B.
  Source: Archives of Ophthalmology. 2001 February; 119(2): 306-7.
  http://www.ncbi.nlm.nih.gov/entrez/query.fcgi?cmd=Retrieve&db=pubmed&dopt=Abstract&list_uids=11177002

- **Bilateral optic nerve sheath enhancement from giant cell arteritis.**
  Author(s): Morgenstern KE, Ellis BD, Schochet SS, Linberg JV.
  Source: The Journal of Rheumatology. 2003 March; 30(3): 625-7.
  http://www.ncbi.nlm.nih.gov/entrez/query.fcgi?cmd=Retrieve&db=pubmed&dopt=Abstract&list_uids=12610827

- **Bilateral percutaneous balloon angioplasty of the axillary arteries in a patient with giant cell arteritis and upper extremity ischemic symptoms not responsive to corticosteroids.**
  Author(s): Dellaripa PF, Eisenhauer AC.
  Source: The Journal of Rheumatology. 1998 July; 25(7): 1429-33.
  http://www.ncbi.nlm.nih.gov/entrez/query.fcgi?cmd=Retrieve&db=pubmed&dopt=Abstract&list_uids=9676780

- **Bilateral scalp necrosis with giant cell arteritis.**
  Author(s): Matsushima M, Yamanaka K, Mori H, Murakami T, Hakamada A, Isoda K, Mizutani H.
  Source: The Journal of Dermatology. 2003 March; 30(3): 210-5.
  http://www.ncbi.nlm.nih.gov/entrez/query.fcgi?cmd=Retrieve&db=pubmed&dopt=Abstract&list_uids=12692357

- **Bilateral superficial femoral giant cell arteritis.**
  Author(s): Tarnoff JF, Pearlman E, Balkoura MH, Venkataraman M.
  Source: The Journal of Cardiovascular Surgery. 1990 May-June; 31(3): 375-9.
  http://www.ncbi.nlm.nih.gov/entrez/query.fcgi?cmd=Retrieve&db=pubmed&dopt=Abstract&list_uids=2196269

- **Bilateral temporal artery biopsies in giant cell arteritis.**
  Author(s): Lessell S.
  Source: Journal of Neuro-Ophthalmology : the Official Journal of the North American Neuro-Ophthalmology Society. 2000 September; 20(3): 220-1.
  http://www.ncbi.nlm.nih.gov/entrez/query.fcgi?cmd=Retrieve&db=pubmed&dopt=Abstract&list_uids=11001200

- **Bilateral vertebral artery occlusion resulting from giant cell arteritis: report of 3 cases and review of the literature.**
  Author(s): Ruegg S, Engelter S, Jeanneret C, Hetzel A, Probst A, Steck AJ, Lyrer P.
  Source: Medicine; Analytical Reviews of General Medicine, Neurology, Psychiatry, Dermatology, and Pediatrics. 2003 January; 82(1): 1-12. Review.
  http://www.ncbi.nlm.nih.gov/entrez/query.fcgi?cmd=Retrieve&db=pubmed&dopt=Abstract&list_uids=12544706

- **Biliary ultrastructural changes in the liver in a case of giant cell arteritis.**
  Author(s): Achar KN, al-Alousi SS, Patrick JP.
  Source: British Journal of Rheumatology. 1994 February; 33(2): 161-4.
  http://www.ncbi.nlm.nih.gov/entrez/query.fcgi?cmd=Retrieve&db=pubmed&dopt=Abstract&list_uids=8162483

- **Biopsy-negative giant cell arteritis: clinical spectrum and predictive factors for positive temporal artery biopsy.**
  Author(s): Gonzalez-Gay MA, Garcia-Porrua C, Llorca J, Gonzalez-Louzao C, Rodriguez-Ledo P.
  Source: Seminars in Arthritis and Rheumatism. 2001 February; 30(4): 249-56.
  http://www.ncbi.nlm.nih.gov/entrez/query.fcgi?cmd=Retrieve&db=pubmed&dopt=Abstract&list_uids=11182025

- **Blindness with a normal erythrocyte sedimentation rate in giant cell arteritis.**
  Author(s): Ellis JD, Munro P, McGettrick P.
  Source: Br J Hosp Med. 1994 October 5-18; 52(7): 358-9. No Abstract Available.
  http://www.ncbi.nlm.nih.gov/entrez/query.fcgi?cmd=Retrieve&db=pubmed&dopt=Abstract&list_uids=7858819

- **Bone mineral content of the third lumbar vertebra during 18 months of prednisolone treatment for giant cell arteritis.**
  Author(s): Nordborg E, Hansson T, Jonson R, Szucs J, Bengtsson BA.
  Source: Clinical Rheumatology. 1993 December; 12(4): 455-60.
  http://www.ncbi.nlm.nih.gov/entrez/query.fcgi?cmd=Retrieve&db=pubmed&dopt=Abstract&list_uids=8124904

- **Bony skull neoplasms masquerading as giant cell arteritis.**
  Author(s): Thomas J, Morris IM, Mattingly PC.
  Source: Hosp Med. 2002 February; 63(2): 114. No Abstract Available.
  http://www.ncbi.nlm.nih.gov/entrez/query.fcgi?cmd=Retrieve&db=pubmed&dopt=Abstract&list_uids=11902084

- **Brachial plexopathy as a presenting symptom of giant cell arteritis.**
  Author(s): Chowdhry IA, Sinha J, Barland P.
  Source: The Journal of Rheumatology. 2002 December; 29(12): 2653-7. Review.
  http://www.ncbi.nlm.nih.gov/entrez/query.fcgi?cmd=Retrieve&db=pubmed&dopt=Abstract&list_uids=12465169

- **Branch retinal artery occlusion as the initial sign of giant cell arteritis.**
  Author(s): Fineman MS, Savino PJ, Federman JL, Eagle RC Jr.
  Source: American Journal of Ophthalmology. 1996 September; 122(3): 428-30.
  http://www.ncbi.nlm.nih.gov/entrez/query.fcgi?cmd=Retrieve&db=pubmed&dopt=Abstract&list_uids=8794719

- **Case 58: giant cell arteritis.**
  Author(s): Lockhart ME, Robbin ML.
  Source: Radiology. 2003 May; 227(2): 512-5.
  http://www.ncbi.nlm.nih.gov/entrez/query.fcgi?cmd=Retrieve&db=pubmed&dopt=Abstract&list_uids=12732702

- **Case number 24: scalp necrosis in giant cell arteritis.**
  Author(s): Khattak FH.
  Source: Annals of the Rheumatic Diseases. 2002 July; 61(7): 590.
  http://www.ncbi.nlm.nih.gov/entrez/query.fcgi?cmd=Retrieve&db=pubmed&dopt=Abstract&list_uids=12079897

- **Case report: acute spontaneous Achilles tendon rupture in a patient with giant cell arteritis.**
  Author(s): Bunch TJ, Welsh GA, Miller DV, Santhi VS.
  Source: Ann Clin Lab Sci. 2003 Summer; 33(3): 326-8.
  http://www.ncbi.nlm.nih.gov/entrez/query.fcgi?cmd=Retrieve&db=pubmed&dopt=Abstract&list_uids=12956450

- **Cavernous sinus syndrome due to vaccination-induced giant cell arteritis.**
  Author(s): Finsterer J, Artner C, Kladosek A, Kalchmayr R, Redtenbacher S.
  Source: Archives of Internal Medicine. 2001 April 9; 161(7): 1008-9.
  http://www.ncbi.nlm.nih.gov/entrez/query.fcgi?cmd=Retrieve&db=pubmed&dopt=Abstract&list_uids=11295966

- **Cerebral infarction due to giant cell arteritis-three case reports.**
  Author(s): Hu Z, Yang Q, Yang L, Li J, Tang J, Zhang H.
  Source: Angiology. 2004 March-April; 55(2): 227-31.
  http://www.ncbi.nlm.nih.gov/entrez/query.fcgi?cmd=Retrieve&db=pubmed&dopt=Abstract&list_uids=15026881

- **Cervical radiculopathy as a manifestation of giant cell arteritis.**
  Author(s): Soubrier M, Dubost JJ, Tournadre A, Deffond D, Clavelou P, Ristori JM.
  Source: Joint, Bone, Spine : Revue Du Rhumatisme. 2002 May; 69(3): 316-8. Review.
  http://www.ncbi.nlm.nih.gov/entrez/query.fcgi?cmd=Retrieve&db=pubmed&dopt=Abstract&list_uids=12102280

- Characteristics of patients presenting with central retinal artery occlusion with and without giant cell arteritis.
  Author(s): Connolly BP, Krishnan A, Shah GK, Whelan J, Brown GC, Eagle RC Jr, Shakin EP.
  Source: Can J Ophthalmol. 2000 December; 35(7): 379-84.
  http://www.ncbi.nlm.nih.gov/entrez/query.fcgi?cmd=Retrieve&db=pubmed&dopt=Abstract&list_uids=11192446

- Chorea--a presenting feature of giant cell arteritis.
  Author(s): Haq N, Shah IA.
  Source: J Pak Med Assoc. 1996 November; 46(11): 263-4. No Abstract Available.
  http://www.ncbi.nlm.nih.gov/entrez/query.fcgi?cmd=Retrieve&db=pubmed&dopt=Abstract&list_uids=9000823

- Choroidal nonperfusion in giant cell arteritis.
  Author(s): Quillen DA, Cantore WA, Schwartz SR, Brod RD, Sassani JW.
  Source: American Journal of Ophthalmology. 1993 August 15; 116(2): 171-5.
  http://www.ncbi.nlm.nih.gov/entrez/query.fcgi?cmd=Retrieve&db=pubmed&dopt=Abstract&list_uids=8352301

- Circulating CD8+ T cells in polymyalgia rheumatica and giant cell arteritis: a review.
  Author(s): Martinez-Taboada VM, Blanco R, Fito C, Pacheco MJ, Delgado-Rodriguez M, Rodriguez-Valverde V.
  Source: Seminars in Arthritis and Rheumatism. 2001 February; 30(4): 257-71. Review.
  http://www.ncbi.nlm.nih.gov/entrez/query.fcgi?cmd=Retrieve&db=pubmed&dopt=Abstract&list_uids=11182026

- Clinical features in patients with permanent visual loss due to biopsy-proven giant cell arteritis.
  Author(s): Font C, Cid MC, Coll-Vinent B, Lopez-Soto A, Grau JM.
  Source: British Journal of Rheumatology. 1997 February; 36(2): 251-4.
  http://www.ncbi.nlm.nih.gov/entrez/query.fcgi?cmd=Retrieve&db=pubmed&dopt=Abstract&list_uids=9133940

- Clues to the pathogenesis of giant cell arteritis from the study of the vessel wall.
  Author(s): Bjornsson J.
  Source: Arthritis Care and Research : the Official Journal of the Arthritis Health Professions Association. 2000 October; 13(5): 249-51.
  http://www.ncbi.nlm.nih.gov/entrez/query.fcgi?cmd=Retrieve&db=pubmed&dopt=Abstract&list_uids=14635291

- Coagulation and fibrinolysis in inflammatory bowel disease and in giant cell arteritis.
  Author(s): Vrij AA, Rijken J, van Wersch JW, Stockbrugger RW.
  Source: Pathophysiology of Haemostasis and Thrombosis. 2003 March-April; 33(2): 75-83.
  http://www.ncbi.nlm.nih.gov/entrez/query.fcgi?cmd=Retrieve&db=pubmed&dopt=Abstract&list_uids=14624048

- **Color Doppler sonography of the temporal arteries in giant cell arteritis and polymyalgia rheumatica.**
  Author(s): Lauwerys BR, Puttemans T, Houssiau FA, Devogelaer JP.
  Source: The Journal of Rheumatology. 1997 August; 24(8): 1570-4.
  http://www.ncbi.nlm.nih.gov/entrez/query.fcgi?cmd=Retrieve&db=pubmed&dopt=Abstract&list_uids=9263153

- **Color duplex ultrasonography in large-vessel giant cell arteritis.**
  Author(s): Schmidt WA, Kraft HE, Borkowski A, Gromnica-Ihle EJ.
  Source: Scandinavian Journal of Rheumatology. 1999; 28(6): 374-6.
  http://www.ncbi.nlm.nih.gov/entrez/query.fcgi?cmd=Retrieve&db=pubmed&dopt=Abstract&list_uids=10665744

- **Colour duplex ultrasonography in the management of giant cell arteritis.**
  Author(s): Nicoletti G, Ciancio G, Tardi S, Olivieri I.
  Source: Clinical Rheumatology. 2003 December; 22(6): 508-9. Epub 2003 November 05.
  http://www.ncbi.nlm.nih.gov/entrez/query.fcgi?cmd=Retrieve&db=pubmed&dopt=Abstract&list_uids=14677048

- **Comparison between color duplex ultrasonography and histology of the temporal artery in cranial arteritis (giant cell arteritis).**
  Author(s): Schmidt D, Hetzel A, Reinhard M, Auw-Haedrich C.
  Source: European Journal of Medical Research. 2003 January 28; 8(1): 1-7.
  http://www.ncbi.nlm.nih.gov/entrez/query.fcgi?cmd=Retrieve&db=pubmed&dopt=Abstract&list_uids=12578748

- **Concordance of bilateral temporal artery biopsy in giant cell arteritis.**
  Author(s): Pless M, Rizzo JF 3rd, Lamkin JC, Lessell S.
  Source: Journal of Neuro-Ophthalmology : the Official Journal of the North American Neuro-Ophthalmology Society. 2000 September; 20(3): 216-8.
  http://www.ncbi.nlm.nih.gov/entrez/query.fcgi?cmd=Retrieve&db=pubmed&dopt=Abstract&list_uids=11001198

- **Correlation of the topographical arrangement and the functional pattern of tissue-infiltrating macrophages in giant cell arteritis.**
  Author(s): Weyand CM, Wagner AD, Bjornsson J, Goronzy JJ.
  Source: The Journal of Clinical Investigation. 1996 October 1; 98(7): 1642-9.
  http://www.ncbi.nlm.nih.gov/entrez/query.fcgi?cmd=Retrieve&db=pubmed&dopt=Abstract&list_uids=8833914

- **Corticotropin releasing hormone promoter polymorphisms in giant cell arteritis and polymyalgia rheumatica.**
  Author(s): Gonzalez-Gay MA, Hajeer AH, Dababneh A, Garcia-Porrua C, Amoli MM, Thomson W, Ollier WE.
  Source: Clin Exp Rheumatol. 2002 March-April; 20(2): 133-8.
  http://www.ncbi.nlm.nih.gov/entrez/query.fcgi?cmd=Retrieve&db=pubmed&dopt=Abstract&list_uids=12051390

- **Deflazacort versus prednisone in patients with giant cell arteritis: effects on bone mass loss.**
  Author(s): Cacoub P, Chemlal K, Khalifa P, Wechsler B, De Gennes C, Belmatoug N, Cohen P, Ziza JM, Verdoncq B, Piette JC.
  Source: The Journal of Rheumatology. 2001 November; 28(11): 2474-9.
  http://www.ncbi.nlm.nih.gov/entrez/query.fcgi?cmd=Retrieve&db=pubmed&dopt=Abstract&list_uids=11708421

- **Dendritic cells co-localize with activated CD4+ T cells in giant cell arteritis.**
  Author(s): Wagner AD, Wittkop U, Prahst A, Schmidt WA, Gromnica-Ihle E, Vorpahl K, Hudson AP, Zeidler H.
  Source: Clin Exp Rheumatol. 2003 March-April; 21(2): 185-92.
  http://www.ncbi.nlm.nih.gov/entrez/query.fcgi?cmd=Retrieve&db=pubmed&dopt=Abstract&list_uids=12747272

- **Detection of parvovirus B19 DNA by polymerase chain reaction in giant cell arteritis: a case-control study.**
  Author(s): Salvarani C, Farnetti E, Casali B, Nicoli D, Wenlan L, Bajocchi G, Macchioni P, Lo Scocco G, Grazia Catanoso M, Boiardi L, Cantini F.
  Source: Arthritis and Rheumatism. 2002 November; 46(11): 3099-101.
  http://www.ncbi.nlm.nih.gov/entrez/query.fcgi?cmd=Retrieve&db=pubmed&dopt=Abstract&list_uids=12428256

- **Detection of posterior ischemic optic neuropathy due to giant cell arteritis with magnetic resonance imaging.**
  Author(s): Lopez JM, Nazabal ER, Muniz AM, Rey del Corral P.
  Source: European Neurology. 2001; 46(2): 109-10.
  http://www.ncbi.nlm.nih.gov/entrez/query.fcgi?cmd=Retrieve&db=pubmed&dopt=Abstract&list_uids=11528166

- **Detection of varicella zoster virus DNA in some patients with giant cell arteritis.**
  Author(s): Mitchell BM, Font RL.
  Source: Investigative Ophthalmology & Visual Science. 2001 October; 42(11): 2572-7.
  http://www.ncbi.nlm.nih.gov/entrez/query.fcgi?cmd=Retrieve&db=pubmed&dopt=Abstract&list_uids=11581201

- **Deterioration of giant cell arteritis with corticosteroid therapy.**
  Author(s): Staunton H, Stafford F, Leader M, O'Riordain D.
  Source: Archives of Neurology. 2000 April; 57(4): 581-4. Review.
  http://www.ncbi.nlm.nih.gov/entrez/query.fcgi?cmd=Retrieve&db=pubmed&dopt=Abstract&list_uids=10768635

- **Diagnoses not to be missed: giant cell arteritis.**
  Author(s): Mulley GP.
  Source: Br J Hosp Med. 1982 April; 27(4): 413-4, 416. No Abstract Available.
  http://www.ncbi.nlm.nih.gov/entrez/query.fcgi?cmd=Retrieve&db=pubmed&dopt=Abstract&list_uids=7074276

- **Diagnosing and managing polymyalgia rheumatica and temporal arteritis. Urgency in giving steroids in giant cell arteritis is still not widely appreciated.**
  Author(s): Freeman AG.
  Source: Bmj (Clinical Research Ed.). 1997 August 30; 315(7107): 549-50.
  http://www.ncbi.nlm.nih.gov/entrez/query.fcgi?cmd=Retrieve&db=pubmed&dopt=Abstract&list_uids=9329328

- **Differential behavior of coagulation factor XIII in patients with inflammatory bowel disease and in patients with giant cell arteritis.**
  Author(s): Vrij AA, Rijken J, van Wersch JW, Stockbrugger RW.
  Source: Haemostasis. 1999 November-December; 29(6): 326-35.
  http://www.ncbi.nlm.nih.gov/entrez/query.fcgi?cmd=Retrieve&db=pubmed&dopt=Abstract&list_uids=10844406

- **Diplopia, ptosis, and hepatitis as presenting signs and symptoms of giant cell arteritis.**
  Author(s): Killer HE, Holtz DJ, Kaiser HJ, Laeng RH.
  Source: The British Journal of Ophthalmology. 2000 November; 84(11): 1319-20.
  http://www.ncbi.nlm.nih.gov/entrez/query.fcgi?cmd=Retrieve&db=pubmed&dopt=Abstract&list_uids=11203169

- **Disease pattern in cranial and large-vessel giant cell arteritis.**
  Author(s): Brack A, Martinez-Taboada V, Stanson A, Goronzy JJ, Weyand CM.
  Source: Arthritis and Rheumatism. 1999 February; 42(2): 311-7.
  http://www.ncbi.nlm.nih.gov/entrez/query.fcgi?cmd=Retrieve&db=pubmed&dopt=Abstract&list_uids=10025926

- **Disease patterns and tissue cytokine profiles in giant cell arteritis.**
  Author(s): Weyand CM, Tetzlaff N, Bjornsson J, Brack A, Younge B, Goronzy JJ.
  Source: Arthritis and Rheumatism. 1997 January; 40(1): 19-26.
  http://www.ncbi.nlm.nih.gov/entrez/query.fcgi?cmd=Retrieve&db=pubmed&dopt=Abstract&list_uids=9008596

- **Disparate results in studies of methotrexate plus corticosteroids in the treatment of giant cell arteritis: comment on the article by Hoffman et al.**
  Author(s): Jover JA, Hernandez-Garcia C, Morado IC, Vargas E, Banares A, Fernandez-Gutierrez B.
  Source: Arthritis and Rheumatism. 2003 April; 48(4): 1158-9.
  http://www.ncbi.nlm.nih.gov/entrez/query.fcgi?cmd=Retrieve&db=pubmed&dopt=Abstract&list_uids=12687561

- **Distinct vascular lesions in giant cell arteritis share identical T cell clonotypes.**
  Author(s): Weyand CM, Schonberger J, Oppitz U, Hunder NN, Hicok KC, Goronzy JJ.
  Source: The Journal of Experimental Medicine. 1994 March 1; 179(3): 951-60.
  http://www.ncbi.nlm.nih.gov/entrez/query.fcgi?cmd=Retrieve&db=pubmed&dopt=Abstract&list_uids=8113687

- **Distribution of HLA-DRB1 alleles of patients with polymyalgia rheumatica and giant cell arteritis in a Mediterranean population.**
  Author(s): Combe B, Sany J, Le Quellec A, Clot J, Eliaou JF.
  Source: The Journal of Rheumatology. 1998 January; 25(1): 94-8.
  http://www.ncbi.nlm.nih.gov/entrez/query.fcgi?cmd=Retrieve&db=pubmed&dopt=Abstract&list_uids=9458210

- **Domains of health-related quality of life important to patients with giant cell arteritis.**
  Author(s): Hellmann DB, Uhlfelder ML, Stone JH, Jenckes MW, Cid MC, Guillevin L, Moreland L, Dellaripa PF, Hoffman GS, Merkel PA, Spiera R, Brown L, Hernandez-Rodriguez J, Rubin HR.
  Source: Arthritis and Rheumatism. 2003 December 15; 49(6): 819-25.
  http://www.ncbi.nlm.nih.gov/entrez/query.fcgi?cmd=Retrieve&db=pubmed&dopt=Abstract&list_uids=14673969

- **Doppler ultrasonography in giant cell arteritis.**
  Author(s): Steigerwalt RD Jr, Cesarone MR, Laurora G, Belcaro G, De Sanctis MT, Incandela L, Christopoulos V.
  Source: International Angiology : a Journal of the International Union of Angiology. 1994 December; 13(4): 286-9.
  http://www.ncbi.nlm.nih.gov/entrez/query.fcgi?cmd=Retrieve&db=pubmed&dopt=Abstract&list_uids=7790746

- **Doppler ultrasonography in the diagnosis of giant cell arteritis.**
  Author(s): Schmidt WA.
  Source: Clin Exp Rheumatol. 2000 July-August; 18(4 Suppl 20): S40-2. Review.
  http://www.ncbi.nlm.nih.gov/entrez/query.fcgi?cmd=Retrieve&db=pubmed&dopt=Abstract&list_uids=10948760

- **Dysarthria associated with giant cell arteritis.**
  Author(s): Lee CC, Su WW, Hunder GG.
  Source: The Journal of Rheumatology. 1999 April; 26(4): 931-2.
  http://www.ncbi.nlm.nih.gov/entrez/query.fcgi?cmd=Retrieve&db=pubmed&dopt=Abstract&list_uids=10229420

- **Effect of prior steroid treatment on temporal artery biopsy findings in giant cell arteritis.**
  Author(s): Ray-Chaudhuri N, Kine DA, Tijani SO, Parums DV, Cartlidge N, Strong NP, Dayan MR.
  Source: The British Journal of Ophthalmology. 2002 May; 86(5): 530-2.
  http://www.ncbi.nlm.nih.gov/entrez/query.fcgi?cmd=Retrieve&db=pubmed&dopt=Abstract&list_uids=11973248

- **Efficacy of unilateral versus bilateral temporal artery biopsies for the diagnosis of giant cell arteritis.**
  Author(s): Ball J, Malhotra R.
  Source: American Journal of Ophthalmology. 2000 April; 129(4): 559-60.
  http://www.ncbi.nlm.nih.gov/entrez/query.fcgi?cmd=Retrieve&db=pubmed&dopt=Abstract&list_uids=10858149

- **Efficacy of unilateral versus bilateral temporal artery biopsies for the diagnosis of giant cell arteritis.**
  Author(s): Lee AG.
  Source: American Journal of Ophthalmology. 2000 January; 129(1): 118-9.
  http://www.ncbi.nlm.nih.gov/entrez/query.fcgi?cmd=Retrieve&db=pubmed&dopt=Abstract&list_uids=10653435

- **Efficacy of unilateral versus bilateral temporal artery biopsies for the diagnosis of giant cell arteritis.**
  Author(s): Boyev LR, Miller NR, Green WR.
  Source: American Journal of Ophthalmology. 1999 August; 128(2): 211-5.
  http://www.ncbi.nlm.nih.gov/entrez/query.fcgi?cmd=Retrieve&db=pubmed&dopt=Abstract&list_uids=10458178

- **Elastase derived elastin peptides: putative autoimmune targets in giant cell arteritis.**
  Author(s): Gillot JM, Masy E, Davril M, Hachulla E, Hatron PY, Devulder B, Dessaint JP.
  Source: The Journal of Rheumatology. 1997 April; 24(4): 677-82.
  http://www.ncbi.nlm.nih.gov/entrez/query.fcgi?cmd=Retrieve&db=pubmed&dopt=Abstract&list_uids=9101501

- **Elastolytic activity of human monocytes. With special reference to rheumatoid arthritis and giant cell arteritis.**
  Author(s): Jensen HS.
  Source: Dan Med Bull. 1993 March; 40(1): 100-10. Review. No Abstract Available.
  http://www.ncbi.nlm.nih.gov/entrez/query.fcgi?cmd=Retrieve&db=pubmed&dopt=Abstract&list_uids=8472593

- **Elevated levels of 92-kd type IV collagenase (matrix metalloproteinase 9) in giant cell arteritis.**
  Author(s): Sorbi D, French DL, Nuovo GJ, Kew RR, Arbeit LA, Gruber BL.
  Source: Arthritis and Rheumatism. 1996 October; 39(10): 1747-53.
  http://www.ncbi.nlm.nih.gov/entrez/query.fcgi?cmd=Retrieve&db=pubmed&dopt=Abstract&list_uids=8843867

- **Enalapril-induced vasculitis resembling rheumatoid arthritis, lupus, sicca syndrome, and giant cell arteritis.**
  Author(s): Berthelot JM, Moreau A, Glemarec J, Mussini JM, Maugars Y, Prost A.
  Source: Rev Rhum Engl Ed. 1997 June; 64(6): 421-3.
  http://www.ncbi.nlm.nih.gov/entrez/query.fcgi?cmd=Retrieve&db=pubmed&dopt=Abstract&list_uids=9513617

- **Endothelial nitric oxide synthase gene polymorphisms in giant cell arteritis.**
  Author(s): Salvarani C, Casali B, Nicoli D, Farnetti E, Macchioni P, Catanoso MG, Chen Q, Bajocchi G, Boiardi L.
  Source: Arthritis and Rheumatism. 2003 November; 48(11): 3219-23.
  http://www.ncbi.nlm.nih.gov/entrez/query.fcgi?cmd=Retrieve&db=pubmed&dopt=Abstract&list_uids=14613286

- **Endothelial nitric oxide synthase haplotype associations in biopsy-proven giant cell arteritis.**
  Author(s): Amoli MM, Garcia-Porrua C, Llorca J, Ollier WE, Gonzalez-Gay MA.
  Source: The Journal of Rheumatology. 2003 September; 30(9): 2019-22.
  http://www.ncbi.nlm.nih.gov/entrez/query.fcgi?cmd=Retrieve&db=pubmed&dopt=Abstract&list_uids=12966609

- **Endovascular repair of thoracic aortic aneurysm and intramural hematoma in giant cell arteritis.**
  Author(s): Engelke C, Sandhu C, Morgan RA, Belli AM.
  Source: Journal of Vascular and Interventional Radiology : Jvir. 2002 June; 13(6): 625-9.
  http://www.ncbi.nlm.nih.gov/entrez/query.fcgi?cmd=Retrieve&db=pubmed&dopt=Abstract&list_uids=12050304

- **Epidemiology of biopsy proven giant cell arteritis in northwestern Spain: trend over an 18 year period.**
  Author(s): Gonzalez-Gay MA, Garcia-Porrua C, Rivas MJ, Rodriguez-Ledo P, Llorca J.
  Source: Annals of the Rheumatic Diseases. 2001 April; 60(4): 367-71.
  http://www.ncbi.nlm.nih.gov/entrez/query.fcgi?cmd=Retrieve&db=pubmed&dopt=Abstract&list_uids=11247867

- **Epidemiology of biopsy-positive giant cell arteritis: an overview.**
  Author(s): Nordborg E.
  Source: Clin Exp Rheumatol. 2000 July-August; 18(4 Suppl 20): S15-7. Review.
  http://www.ncbi.nlm.nih.gov/entrez/query.fcgi?cmd=Retrieve&db=pubmed&dopt=Abstract&list_uids=10948751

- **Epidemiology of giant cell arteritis.**
  Author(s): Bengtsson BA.
  Source: Baillieres Clin Rheumatol. 1991 December; 5(3): 379-85. Review. No Abstract Available.
  http://www.ncbi.nlm.nih.gov/entrez/query.fcgi?cmd=Retrieve&db=pubmed&dopt=Abstract&list_uids=1807816

- **Estrogen receptor alpha in giant cell arteritis: a molecular genetic study.**
  Author(s): Petursdottir V, Moslemi AR, Persson M, Nordborg E, Nordborg C.
  Source: Clin Exp Rheumatol. 2001 May-June; 19(3): 297-302.
  http://www.ncbi.nlm.nih.gov/entrez/query.fcgi?cmd=Retrieve&db=pubmed&dopt=Abstract&list_uids=11407083

- **Estrogen receptors in giant cell arteritis. An immunocytochemical, western blot and RT-PCR study.**
  Author(s): Petursdottir V, Nordborg E, Moraghebi N, Persson M, Nordborg C.
  Source: Clin Exp Rheumatol. 1999 November-December; 17(6): 671-7.
  http://www.ncbi.nlm.nih.gov/entrez/query.fcgi?cmd=Retrieve&db=pubmed&dopt=Abstract&list_uids=10609065

- **Experience with infliximab (anti-TNF alpha monoclonal antibody) as monotherapy for giant cell arteritis.**
  Author(s): Andonopoulos AP, Meimaris N, Daoussis D, Bounas A, Giannopoulos G.
  Source: Annals of the Rheumatic Diseases. 2003 November; 62(11): 1116.
  http://www.ncbi.nlm.nih.gov/entrez/query.fcgi?cmd=Retrieve&db=pubmed&dopt=Abstract&list_uids=14583578

- **Extensive scalp necrosis and subepicranial abscess in a patient with giant cell arteritis.**
  Author(s): Smitz S, Van Damme H.
  Source: Journal of the American Geriatrics Society. 2004 January; 52(1): 165-6.
  http://www.ncbi.nlm.nih.gov/entrez/query.fcgi?cmd=Retrieve&db=pubmed&dopt=Abstract&list_uids=14687340

- **Extracranial giant cell arteritis restricted to the small bowel.**
  Author(s): Krant JD, Ross JM.
  Source: Arthritis and Rheumatism. 1992 May; 35(5): 603-4.
  http://www.ncbi.nlm.nih.gov/entrez/query.fcgi?cmd=Retrieve&db=pubmed&dopt=Abstract&list_uids=1575796

- **Extracranial giant cell arteritis.**
  Author(s): Evans DJ, Wilkins MJ, Wazir JF, Rosin D.
  Source: Journal of the Royal College of Surgeons of Edinburgh. 1998 June; 43(3): 207-8.
  http://www.ncbi.nlm.nih.gov/entrez/query.fcgi?cmd=Retrieve&db=pubmed&dopt=Abstract&list_uids=9654889

- **F18-FDG-PET as a helpful tool in the diagnosis of giant cell arteritis.**
  Author(s): Brodmann M, Passath A, Aigner R, Seinost G, Stark G, Pilger E.
  Source: Rheumatology (Oxford, England). 2003 October; 42(10): 1264-6.
  http://www.ncbi.nlm.nih.gov/entrez/query.fcgi?cmd=Retrieve&db=pubmed&dopt=Abstract&list_uids=14508046

- **Facial edema and giant cell arteritis.**
  Author(s): Plantin P, Caplanne D, Rosenberg F, Le Parc JM.
  Source: Rev Rhum Engl Ed. 1996 February; 63(2): 145-7. Review.
  http://www.ncbi.nlm.nih.gov/entrez/query.fcgi?cmd=Retrieve&db=pubmed&dopt=Abstract&list_uids=8689287

- **Facial pain and giant cell arteritis.**
  Author(s): Gonzalez-Gay MA, Garcia-Porrua C, Gonzalez-Roson O.
  Source: The Journal of Rheumatology. 1998 June; 25(6): 1242-3.
  http://www.ncbi.nlm.nih.gov/entrez/query.fcgi?cmd=Retrieve&db=pubmed&dopt=Abstract&list_uids=9632096

- **Facial swelling and giant cell arteritis.**
  Author(s): Cohen MD, Ginsburg WW, Allen GL.
  Source: The Journal of Rheumatology. 1982 March-April; 9(2): 325-7.
  http://www.ncbi.nlm.nih.gov/entrez/query.fcgi?cmd=Retrieve&db=pubmed&dopt=Abstract&list_uids=7097696

- **Factor VIII-von Willebrand factor in giant cell arteritis and polymyalgia rheumatica.**
  Author(s): Persellin ST, Daniels TM, Rings LJ, Kazmier FJ, Bowie EJ, Hunder GG.
  Source: Mayo Clinic Proceedings. 1985 July; 60(7): 457-62.
  http://www.ncbi.nlm.nih.gov/entrez/query.fcgi?cmd=Retrieve&db=pubmed&dopt=Abstract&list_uids=3925247

- **Familial aggregation of polymyalgia rheumatica and giant cell arteritis: genetic and T cell repertoire analysis.**
  Author(s): Bartolome MJ, Martinez-Taboda VM, Lopez-Hoyos M, Blanco R, Rodriguez-Valverde V.
  Source: Clin Exp Rheumatol. 2001 May-June; 19(3): 259-64.
  http://www.ncbi.nlm.nih.gov/entrez/query.fcgi?cmd=Retrieve&db=pubmed&dopt=Abstract&list_uids=11407077

- **Familial association of giant cell arteritis. A case report and brief review.**
  Author(s): Granato JE, Abben RP, May WS.
  Source: Archives of Internal Medicine. 1981 January; 141(1): 115-7.
  http://www.ncbi.nlm.nih.gov/entrez/query.fcgi?cmd=Retrieve&db=pubmed&dopt=Abstract&list_uids=7447573

- **Familial giant cell arteritis and polymyalgia rheumatica: aggregation in 2 families.**
  Author(s): Fietta P, Manganelli P, Zanetti A, Neri TM.
  Source: The Journal of Rheumatology. 2002 July; 29(7): 1551-5.
  http://www.ncbi.nlm.nih.gov/entrez/query.fcgi?cmd=Retrieve&db=pubmed&dopt=Abstract&list_uids=12136919

- **Familial giant cell arteritis.**
  Author(s): Novak MA, Green WR, Miller NR.
  Source: J Clin Neuroophthalmol. 1986 June; 6(2): 126. No Abstract Available.
  http://www.ncbi.nlm.nih.gov/entrez/query.fcgi?cmd=Retrieve&db=pubmed&dopt=Abstract&list_uids=2942569

- **Familial giant cell arteritis: report of an HLA-typed sibling pair and a review of the literature.**
  Author(s): Wernick R, Davey M, Bonafede P.
  Source: Clin Exp Rheumatol. 1994 January-February; 12(1): 63-6. Review.
  http://www.ncbi.nlm.nih.gov/entrez/query.fcgi?cmd=Retrieve&db=pubmed&dopt=Abstract&list_uids=8162645

- **Fatal renal failure in polymyalgia rheumatica caused by disseminated giant cell arteritis.**
  Author(s): Elling H, Kristensen IB.
  Source: Scandinavian Journal of Rheumatology. 1980; 9(4): 206-8.
  http://www.ncbi.nlm.nih.gov/entrez/query.fcgi?cmd=Retrieve&db=pubmed&dopt=Abstract&list_uids=7455632

- **Fatal varicella-zoster virus antigen-positive giant cell arteritis of the central nervous system.**
  Author(s): Berger TM, Caduff JH, Gebbers JO.
  Source: The Pediatric Infectious Disease Journal. 2000 July; 19(7): 653-6.
  http://www.ncbi.nlm.nih.gov/entrez/query.fcgi?cmd=Retrieve&db=pubmed&dopt=A
  bstract&list_uids=10917225

- **Fatal vertebral giant cell arteritis.**
  Author(s): Sheehan MM, Keohane C, Twomey C.
  Source: Journal of Clinical Pathology. 1993 December; 46(12): 1129-31.
  http://www.ncbi.nlm.nih.gov/entrez/query.fcgi?cmd=Retrieve&db=pubmed&dopt=A
  bstract&list_uids=8282839

- **Female genital tract giant cell arteritis associated with occult temporal arteritis.**
  Author(s): Inanc M, Gul A, Tuzlali S, Buyru F, Konice M, Aral O, Ocal L, Ilhan R, Lie JT.
  Source: The Journal of Rheumatology. 1996 February; 23(2): 393-5.
  http://www.ncbi.nlm.nih.gov/entrez/query.fcgi?cmd=Retrieve&db=pubmed&dopt=A
  bstract&list_uids=8882055

- **First international conference on polymyalgia rheumatica and giant cell arteritis, Prato, Italy. May 25-26, 1999.**
  Author(s): Schirmer M, Calamia KT, Salvarani C.
  Source: The Journal of Rheumatology. 2000 July; 27(7): 1801-3.
  http://www.ncbi.nlm.nih.gov/entrez/query.fcgi?cmd=Retrieve&db=pubmed&dopt=A
  bstract&list_uids=10914874

- **First report of giant cell arteritis--in the Talmud.**
  Author(s): Gurvich TR.
  Source: The Journal of Rheumatology. 1998 April; 25(4): 828.
  http://www.ncbi.nlm.nih.gov/entrez/query.fcgi?cmd=Retrieve&db=pubmed&dopt=A
  bstract&list_uids=9558203

- **Fludeoxyglucose positron emission tomography in the diagnosis of giant cell arteritis.**
  Author(s): Turlakow A, Yeung HW, Pui J, Macapinlac H, Liebovitz E, Rusch V, Goy A, Larson SM.
  Source: Archives of Internal Medicine. 2001 April 9; 161(7): 1003-7.
  http://www.ncbi.nlm.nih.gov/entrez/query.fcgi?cmd=Retrieve&db=pubmed&dopt=A
  bstract&list_uids=11295964

- **Fluorescein angiography in the diagnosis of giant cell arteritis.**
  Author(s): Siatkowski RM, Gass JD, Glaser JS, Smith JL, Schatz NJ, Schiffman J.
  Source: American Journal of Ophthalmology. 1993 January; 115(1): 57-63.
  http://www.ncbi.nlm.nih.gov/entrez/query.fcgi?cmd=Retrieve&db=pubmed&dopt=A
  bstract&list_uids=8420379

- Fluorodeoxyglucose positron emission tomography for the diagnosis of giant cell arteritis.
  Author(s): Famularo G, Minisola G, De Simone C.
  Source: Rheumatology (Oxford, England). 2004 May; 43(5): 679; Author Reply 679-80.
  http://www.ncbi.nlm.nih.gov/entrez/query.fcgi?cmd=Retrieve&db=pubmed&dopt=Abstract&list_uids=15103041

- Functional profile of tissue-infiltrating and circulating CD68+ cells in giant cell arteritis. Evidence for two components of the disease.
  Author(s): Wagner AD, Goronzy JJ, Weyand CM.
  Source: The Journal of Clinical Investigation. 1994 September; 94(3): 1134-40.
  http://www.ncbi.nlm.nih.gov/entrez/query.fcgi?cmd=Retrieve&db=pubmed&dopt=Abstract&list_uids=8083354

- Geographical and genetic factors do not account for significant differences in the clinical spectrum of giant cell arteritis in southern europe.
  Author(s): Gonzalez-Gay MA, Boiardi L, Garcia-Porrua C, Macchioni P, Amor-Dorado JC, Salvarani C.
  Source: The Journal of Rheumatology. 2004 March; 31(3): 520-3.
  http://www.ncbi.nlm.nih.gov/entrez/query.fcgi?cmd=Retrieve&db=pubmed&dopt=Abstract&list_uids=14994398

- Giant cell arteritis (temporal arteritis, cranial arteritis) and a case from Singapore.
  Author(s): Cullen JF, Chan CM, Chuah KL.
  Source: Singapore Med J. 2003 June; 44(6): 306-8.
  http://www.ncbi.nlm.nih.gov/entrez/query.fcgi?cmd=Retrieve&db=pubmed&dopt=Abstract&list_uids=14560864

- Giant cell arteritis and polymyalgia rheumatica.
  Author(s): Hunder GG.
  Source: The Medical Clinics of North America. 1997 January; 81(1): 195-219. Review.
  http://www.ncbi.nlm.nih.gov/entrez/query.fcgi?cmd=Retrieve&db=pubmed&dopt=Abstract&list_uids=9012761

- Giant cell arteritis and polymyalgia rheumatica: clues to early diagnosis.
  Author(s): Dwolatzky T, Sonnenblick M, Nesher G.
  Source: Geriatrics. 1997 June; 52(6): 38-40, 43-4.
  http://www.ncbi.nlm.nih.gov/entrez/query.fcgi?cmd=Retrieve&db=pubmed&dopt=Abstract&list_uids=9194789

- Giant cell arteritis in polymyalgia rheumatica.
  Author(s): Hunder GG.
  Source: The American Journal of Medicine. 1997 June; 102(6): 514-6.
  http://www.ncbi.nlm.nih.gov/entrez/query.fcgi?cmd=Retrieve&db=pubmed&dopt=Abstract&list_uids=9217664

- **Giant cell arteritis involving the lower limbs.**
  Author(s): Dupuy R, Mercie P, Neau D, Longy-Boursier M, Conri C.
  Source: Rev Rhum Engl Ed. 1997 July-September; 64(7-9): 500-3.
  http://www.ncbi.nlm.nih.gov/entrez/query.fcgi?cmd=Retrieve&db=pubmed&dopt=A
  bstract&list_uids=9338933

- **Giant cell arteritis masquerading as squamous cell carcinoma of the skin.**
  Author(s): Assi A, Nischal KK, Uddin J, Thyveetil MD.
  Source: British Journal of Rheumatology. 1997 September; 36(9): 1023-5.
  http://www.ncbi.nlm.nih.gov/entrez/query.fcgi?cmd=Retrieve&db=pubmed&dopt=A
  bstract&list_uids=9376980

- **Giant cell arteritis of the female genital tract.**
  Author(s): Walsh T, Lyons F, Sinha SK, Khawaja N, Harrison M, Boyd W, Couglan M.
  Source: Ir Med J. 2004 January; 97(1): 23. No Abstract Available.
  http://www.ncbi.nlm.nih.gov/entrez/query.fcgi?cmd=Retrieve&db=pubmed&dopt=A
  bstract&list_uids=15055921

- **Giant cell arteritis of the female genital tract.**
  Author(s): Piura B, Wolak A, Rabinovich A, Yanai-Inbar I.
  Source: Clin Exp Obstet Gynecol. 2004; 31(1): 31-3. Review.
  http://www.ncbi.nlm.nih.gov/entrez/query.fcgi?cmd=Retrieve&db=pubmed&dopt=A
  bstract&list_uids=14998183

- **Giant cell arteritis of the uterus: case report and review.**
  Author(s): Ormsby AH, Haskell R.
  Source: Pathology. 1997 May; 29(2): 227-30. Review.
  http://www.ncbi.nlm.nih.gov/entrez/query.fcgi?cmd=Retrieve&db=pubmed&dopt=A
  bstract&list_uids=9213348

- **Giant cell arteritis presenting as a carpal tunnel syndrome.**
  Author(s): Dennis RH 2nd, Ransome JR.
  Source: Journal of the National Medical Association. 1996 August; 88(8): 524-5.
  http://www.ncbi.nlm.nih.gov/entrez/query.fcgi?cmd=Retrieve&db=pubmed&dopt=A
  bstract&list_uids=8803435

- **Giant cell arteritis presenting with oculomotor nerve palsy.**
  Author(s): Bondeson J, Asman P.
  Source: Scandinavian Journal of Rheumatology. 1997; 26(4): 327-8.
  http://www.ncbi.nlm.nih.gov/entrez/query.fcgi?cmd=Retrieve&db=pubmed&dopt=A
  bstract&list_uids=9310116

- **Giant cell arteritis with unusual flow-related neuro-ophthalmologic manifestations.**
  Author(s): Galetta SL, Balcer LJ, Liu GT.
  Source: Neurology. 1997 November; 49(5): 1463-5.
  http://www.ncbi.nlm.nih.gov/entrez/query.fcgi?cmd=Retrieve&db=pubmed&dopt=A
  bstract&list_uids=9371944

- **Giant cell arteritis without clinically evident vascular involvement in a defined population.**
  Author(s): Gonzalez-Gay MA, Garcia-Porrua C, Amor-Dorado JC, Llorca J.
  Source: Arthritis and Rheumatism. 2004 April 15; 51(2): 274-7.
  http://www.ncbi.nlm.nih.gov/entrez/query.fcgi?cmd=Retrieve&db=pubmed&dopt=Abstract&list_uids=15077272

- **Giant cell arteritis, scalp necrosis and myocardial infarction.**
  Author(s): Grant S.
  Source: Internal Medicine Journal. 2004 March; 34(3): 138-9.
  http://www.ncbi.nlm.nih.gov/entrez/query.fcgi?cmd=Retrieve&db=pubmed&dopt=Abstract&list_uids=15030467

- **Giant cell arteritis: diagnosis and management.**
  Author(s): Kachroo A, Tello C, Bais R, Panush RS.
  Source: Bulletin on the Rheumatic Diseases. 1996 August; 45(5): 2-5.
  http://www.ncbi.nlm.nih.gov/entrez/query.fcgi?cmd=Retrieve&db=pubmed&dopt=Abstract&list_uids=8768498

- **Giant cell arteritis: new concepts in pathogenesis and implications for management.**
  Author(s): Weyand CM, Bartley GB.
  Source: American Journal of Ophthalmology. 1997 March; 123(3): 392-5. Review.
  http://www.ncbi.nlm.nih.gov/entrez/query.fcgi?cmd=Retrieve&db=pubmed&dopt=Abstract&list_uids=9063250

- **Giant cell arteritis: strategies in diagnosis and treatment.**
  Author(s): Nordborg E, Nordborg C.
  Source: Current Opinion in Rheumatology. 2004 January; 16(1): 25-30. Review.
  http://www.ncbi.nlm.nih.gov/entrez/query.fcgi?cmd=Retrieve&db=pubmed&dopt=Abstract&list_uids=14673385

- **Giant cell arteritis: validity and reliability of various diagnostic criteria.**
  Author(s): Hayreh SS, Podhajsky PA, Raman R, Zimmerman B.
  Source: American Journal of Ophthalmology. 1997 March; 123(3): 285-96.
  http://www.ncbi.nlm.nih.gov/entrez/query.fcgi?cmd=Retrieve&db=pubmed&dopt=Abstract&list_uids=9063237

- **Giant cell arteritis--a case report.**
  Author(s): Nixon PP, Payne M, Franklin CD.
  Source: British Dental Journal. 1997 October 11; 183(7): 260-2.
  http://www.ncbi.nlm.nih.gov/entrez/query.fcgi?cmd=Retrieve&db=pubmed&dopt=Abstract&list_uids=9364094

- **Heeding clues to giant cell arteritis. Prompt response can prevent vision loss.**
  Author(s): Lichtstein DM, Caceres LR.
  Source: Postgraduate Medicine. 2004 May; 115(5): 91-5.
  http://www.ncbi.nlm.nih.gov/entrez/query.fcgi?cmd=Retrieve&db=pubmed&dopt=Abstract&list_uids=15171082

- **Hemidiaphragm paralysis: a new pulmonary manifestation of giant cell arteritis.**
  Author(s): Hong MK, Hellmann DB.
  Source: The Journal of Rheumatology. 1989 February; 16(2): 253-4.
  http://www.ncbi.nlm.nih.gov/entrez/query.fcgi?cmd=Retrieve&db=pubmed&dopt=A
  bstract&list_uids=2746576

- **Heparin therapy in giant cell arteritis.**
  Author(s): Buono LM, Foroozan R, de Virgiliis M, Savino PJ.
  Source: The British Journal of Ophthalmology. 2004 February; 88(2): 298-301.
  http://www.ncbi.nlm.nih.gov/entrez/query.fcgi?cmd=Retrieve&db=pubmed&dopt=A
  bstract&list_uids=14736795

- **Hepatic fibrin-ring granulomas in giant cell arteritis.**
  Author(s): de Bayser L, Roblot P, Ramassamy A, Silvain C, Levillain P, Becq-Giraudon B.
  Source: Gastroenterology. 1993 July; 105(1): 272-3.
  http://www.ncbi.nlm.nih.gov/entrez/query.fcgi?cmd=Retrieve&db=pubmed&dopt=A
  bstract&list_uids=8514044

- **Herpes zoster ophthalmicus masquerading as giant cell arteritis.**
  Author(s): Chittenden HB, Clearkin LG, Sidky K.
  Source: Br J Hosp Med. 1995 June 21-July 11; 54(1): 49-50. No Abstract Available.
  http://www.ncbi.nlm.nih.gov/entrez/query.fcgi?cmd=Retrieve&db=pubmed&dopt=A
  bstract&list_uids=7551476

- **Herpes zoster vasculitis presenting as giant cell arteritis with bilateral internuclear ophthalmoplegia.**
  Author(s): Al-Abdulla NA, Rismondo V, Minkowski JS, Miller NR.
  Source: American Journal of Ophthalmology. 2002 December; 134(6): 912-4.
  http://www.ncbi.nlm.nih.gov/entrez/query.fcgi?cmd=Retrieve&db=pubmed&dopt=A
  bstract&list_uids=12470766

- **Herpes zoster vasculitis presenting as giant cell arteritis with choroidal infarction.**
  Author(s): Al-Abdulla NA, Kelley JS, Green WR, Miller NR.
  Source: Retina (Philadelphia, Pa.). 2003 August; 23(4): 567-9.
  http://www.ncbi.nlm.nih.gov/entrez/query.fcgi?cmd=Retrieve&db=pubmed&dopt=A
  bstract&list_uids=12972779

- **High circulating leukaemia inhibitory factor (LIF) in patients with giant cell arteritis: independent regulation of LIF and IL-6 under corticosteroid therapy.**
  Author(s): Lecron JC, Roblot P, Chevalier S, Morel F, Alderman E, Gombert J, Gascan H.
  Source: Clinical and Experimental Immunology. 1993 April; 92(1): 23-6.
  http://www.ncbi.nlm.nih.gov/entrez/query.fcgi?cmd=Retrieve&db=pubmed&dopt=A
  bstract&list_uids=8096803

- **High incidence of polymyalgia rheumatica and giant cell arteritis in a Swedish community.**
  Author(s): Noltorp S, Svensson B.
  Source: Clin Exp Rheumatol. 1991 July-August; 9(4): 351-5.
  http://www.ncbi.nlm.nih.gov/entrez/query.fcgi?cmd=Retrieve&db=pubmed&dopt=Abstract&list_uids=1934682

- **HLA-DRB1 alleles in polymyalgia rheumatica, giant cell arteritis, and rheumatoid arthritis.**
  Author(s): Weyand CM, Hunder NN, Hicok KC, Hunder GG, Goronzy JJ.
  Source: Arthritis and Rheumatism. 1994 April; 37(4): 514-20.
  http://www.ncbi.nlm.nih.gov/entrez/query.fcgi?cmd=Retrieve&db=pubmed&dopt=Abstract&list_uids=8147928

- **HLA-DRB1*04 may be a marker of severity in giant cell arteritis.**
  Author(s): Gonzalez-Gay MA, Garcia-Porrua C, Hajeer AH, Dababneh A, Ollier WE.
  Source: Annals of the Rheumatic Diseases. 2000 July; 59(7): 574-5.
  http://www.ncbi.nlm.nih.gov/entrez/query.fcgi?cmd=Retrieve&db=pubmed&dopt=Abstract&list_uids=10950753

- **HLA-DRB1, DQA1, and DQB1 alleles associated with giant cell arteritis in northern Italy.**
  Author(s): Salvarani C, Boiardi L, Mantovani V, Ranzi A, Cantini F, Olivieri I, Viggiani M, Bragliani M, Macchioni P.
  Source: The Journal of Rheumatology. 1999 November; 26(11): 2395-9.
  http://www.ncbi.nlm.nih.gov/entrez/query.fcgi?cmd=Retrieve&db=pubmed&dopt=Abstract&list_uids=10555899

- **Homocysteine levels in polymyalgia rheumatica and giant cell arteritis: influence of corticosteroid therapy.**
  Author(s): Martinez-Taboada VM, Bartolome MJ, Fernandez-Gonzalez MD, Blanco R, Rodriguez-Valverde V, Lopez-Hoyos M.
  Source: Rheumatology (Oxford, England). 2003 September; 42(9): 1055-61. Epub 2003 April 16.
  http://www.ncbi.nlm.nih.gov/entrez/query.fcgi?cmd=Retrieve&db=pubmed&dopt=Abstract&list_uids=12730520

- **Horton giant cell arteritis of the legs. Report of a case.**
  Author(s): Amatucci G, Del Mastro G, Iandoli R.
  Source: The Journal of Cardiovascular Surgery. 1997 June; 38(3): 309-12. Review.
  http://www.ncbi.nlm.nih.gov/entrez/query.fcgi?cmd=Retrieve&db=pubmed&dopt=Abstract&list_uids=9219484

- **Human Parvovirus and giant cell arteritis: a selective arteritic impact?**
  Author(s): Elling H, Olsson AT, Elling P.
  Source: Clin Exp Rheumatol. 2000 July-August; 18(4 Suppl 20): S12-4.
  http://www.ncbi.nlm.nih.gov/entrez/query.fcgi?cmd=Retrieve&db=pubmed&dopt=Abstract&list_uids=10948750

- **Hyperaldosteronism secondary to giant cell arteritis.**
  Author(s): Wrong OM.
  Source: Nephron. 2001 July; 88(3): 286.
  http://www.ncbi.nlm.nih.gov/entrez/query.fcgi?cmd=Retrieve&db=pubmed&dopt=A
  bstract&list_uids=11423767

- **Hypokalemic metabolic alkalosis secondary to giant cell arteritis.**
  Author(s): Justo-Muradas I, Perez-Suarez M, Saracibar E, Sedano E, Perez-Castrillon JL.
  Source: Nephron. 2000 December; 86(4): 524-5.
  http://www.ncbi.nlm.nih.gov/entrez/query.fcgi?cmd=Retrieve&db=pubmed&dopt=A
  bstract&list_uids=11124613

- **Hypothalamic-pituitary-adrenocortical axis function in patients with polymyalgia rheumatica and giant cell arteritis.**
  Author(s): Pacheco MJ, Amado JA, Lopez-Hoyos M, Blanco R, Garcia-Unzueta MT, Rodriguez-Valverde V, Martinez-Taboada VM.
  Source: Seminars in Arthritis and Rheumatism. 2003 February; 32(4): 266-72.
  http://www.ncbi.nlm.nih.gov/entrez/query.fcgi?cmd=Retrieve&db=pubmed&dopt=A
  bstract&list_uids=12621591

- **Hypothyroidism in polymyalgia rheumatica and giant cell arteritis.**
  Author(s): Wiseman P, Stewart K, Rai GS.
  Source: Bmj (Clinical Research Ed.). 1989 March 11; 298(6674): 647-8.
  http://www.ncbi.nlm.nih.gov/entrez/query.fcgi?cmd=Retrieve&db=pubmed&dopt=A
  bstract&list_uids=2496792

- **Hypothyroidism in polymyalgia rheumatica and giant cell arteritis: lack of any association.**
  Author(s): Dasgupta B, Grundy E, Stainer E.
  Source: Bmj (Clinical Research Ed.). 1990 July 14; 301(6743): 96-7.
  http://www.ncbi.nlm.nih.gov/entrez/query.fcgi?cmd=Retrieve&db=pubmed&dopt=A
  bstract&list_uids=2390592

- **Identification of candidate microbial sequences from inflammatory lesion of giant cell arteritis.**
  Author(s): Gordon LK, Goldman M, Sandusky H, Ziv N, Hoffman GS, Goodglick T, Goodglick L.
  Source: Clinical Immunology (Orlando, Fla.). 2004 June; 111(3): 286-96.
  http://www.ncbi.nlm.nih.gov/entrez/query.fcgi?cmd=Retrieve&db=pubmed&dopt=A
  bstract&list_uids=15183149

- **Idiopathic lateral sinus thrombosis mimicking giant cell arteritis.**
  Author(s): Garcia-Porrua C, Vega Andion J, Gonzalez-Gay MA.
  Source: The Journal of Rheumatology. 2001 September; 28(9): 2142-3.
  http://www.ncbi.nlm.nih.gov/entrez/query.fcgi?cmd=Retrieve&db=pubmed&dopt=A
  bstract&list_uids=11550994

- IL-6 promoter polymorphism at position -174 modulates the phenotypic expression of polymyalgia rheumatica in biopsy-proven giant cell arteritis.
  Author(s): Gonzalez-Gay MA, Hajeer AH, Dababneh A, Garcia-Porrua C, Mattey DL, Amoli MM, Thomson W, Ollier WE.
  Source: Clin Exp Rheumatol. 2002 March-April; 20(2): 179-84.
  http://www.ncbi.nlm.nih.gov/entrez/query.fcgi?cmd=Retrieve&db=pubmed&dopt=Abstract&list_uids=12051396

- Imaging of giant cell arteritis: evidence of splenic involvement using FDG positron emission tomography.
  Author(s): De Winter F, Petrovic M, Van de Wiele C, Vogelaers D, Afschrift M, Dierckx RA.
  Source: Clinical Nuclear Medicine. 2000 August; 25(8): 633-4.
  http://www.ncbi.nlm.nih.gov/entrez/query.fcgi?cmd=Retrieve&db=pubmed&dopt=Abstract&list_uids=10944026

- Immediate and long-term outcome of upper extremity balloon angioplasty in giant cell arteritis.
  Author(s): Amann-Vesti BR, Koppensteiner R, Rainoni L, Pfamatter T, Schneider E.
  Source: Journal of Endovascular Therapy : an Official Journal of the International Society of Endovascular Specialists. 2003 April; 10(2): 371-5.
  http://www.ncbi.nlm.nih.gov/entrez/query.fcgi?cmd=Retrieve&db=pubmed&dopt=Abstract&list_uids=12877626

- Immunology and ocular manifestations of giant cell arteritis.
  Author(s): Barchuk WT, Centeno L, Frohman L, Bielory L.
  Source: Ocular Immunology and Inflammation. 1997 June; 5(2): 141-6.
  http://www.ncbi.nlm.nih.gov/entrez/query.fcgi?cmd=Retrieve&db=pubmed&dopt=Abstract&list_uids=9234378

- Implications of thrombocytosis in giant cell arteritis.
  Author(s): Krishna R, Kosmorsky GS.
  Source: American Journal of Ophthalmology. 1997 July; 124(1): 103.
  http://www.ncbi.nlm.nih.gov/entrez/query.fcgi?cmd=Retrieve&db=pubmed&dopt=Abstract&list_uids=9222239

- Incidence and predictors of large-artery complication (aortic aneurysm, aortic dissection, and/or large-artery stenosis) in patients with giant cell arteritis: a population-based study over 50 years.
  Author(s): Nuenninghoff DM, Hunder GG, Christianson TJ, McClelland RL, Matteson EL.
  Source: Arthritis and Rheumatism. 2003 December; 48(12): 3522-31.
  http://www.ncbi.nlm.nih.gov/entrez/query.fcgi?cmd=Retrieve&db=pubmed&dopt=Abstract&list_uids=14674004

- Increased endothelin-1 plasma levels in giant cell arteritis: a report on four patients.
  Author(s): Pache M, Kaiser HJ, Haufschild T, Lubeck P, Flammer J.
  Source: American Journal of Ophthalmology. 2002 January; 133(1): 160-2.
  http://www.ncbi.nlm.nih.gov/entrez/query.fcgi?cmd=Retrieve&db=pubmed&dopt=Abstract&list_uids=11755863

- **Increased mortality due to cardiovascular disease in patients with giant cell arteritis in northern Sweden.**
  Author(s): Uddhammar A, Eriksson AL, Nystrom L, Stenling R, Rantapaa-Dahlqvist S.
  Source: The Journal of Rheumatology. 2002 April; 29(4): 737-42.
  http://www.ncbi.nlm.nih.gov/entrez/query.fcgi?cmd=Retrieve&db=pubmed&dopt=Abstract&list_uids=11950015

- **Infarction of the sigmoid colon secondary to giant cell arteritis.**
  Author(s): Trimble MA, Weisz MA.
  Source: Rheumatology (Oxford, England). 2002 January; 41(1): 108-10.
  http://www.ncbi.nlm.nih.gov/entrez/query.fcgi?cmd=Retrieve&db=pubmed&dopt=Abstract&list_uids=11792890

- **Influence of age, sex, and place of residence on clinical expression of giant cell arteritis in northwest Spain.**
  Author(s): Gonzalez-Gay MA, Garcia-Porrua C, Amor-Dorado JC, Llorca J.
  Source: The Journal of Rheumatology. 2003 July; 30(7): 1548-51.
  http://www.ncbi.nlm.nih.gov/entrez/query.fcgi?cmd=Retrieve&db=pubmed&dopt=Abstract&list_uids=12858456

- **Internuclear ophthalmoplegia and Horner's syndrome due to presumed giant cell arteritis.**
  Author(s): Askari A, Jolobe OM, Shepherd DI.
  Source: Journal of the Royal Society of Medicine. 1993 June; 86(6): 362.
  http://www.ncbi.nlm.nih.gov/entrez/query.fcgi?cmd=Retrieve&db=pubmed&dopt=Abstract&list_uids=8315638

- **Intracranial giant cell arteritis with fatal middle cerebral artery territory infarct.**
  Author(s): Browne L, Hardiman O, O'Dwyer H, Farrell M.
  Source: Clin Neuropathol. 2003 July-August; 22(4): 199-203.
  http://www.ncbi.nlm.nih.gov/entrez/query.fcgi?cmd=Retrieve&db=pubmed&dopt=Abstract&list_uids=12908757

- **Intraoral lesion in giant cell arteritis.**
  Author(s): Kannan R, Allen CM, Ockner SA, Schneider KE.
  Source: Oral Surgery, Oral Medicine, Oral Pathology, Oral Radiology, and Endodontics. 1996 November; 82(5): 473-4.
  http://www.ncbi.nlm.nih.gov/entrez/query.fcgi?cmd=Retrieve&db=pubmed&dopt=Abstract&list_uids=8936508

- **Involvement of peripheral arteries in giant cell arteritis: a color Doppler sonography study.**
  Author(s): Schmidt WA, Natusch A, Moller DE, Vorpahl K, Gromnica-Ihle E.
  Source: Clin Exp Rheumatol. 2002 May-June; 20(3): 309-18.
  http://www.ncbi.nlm.nih.gov/entrez/query.fcgi?cmd=Retrieve&db=pubmed&dopt=Abstract&list_uids=12102466

- **Involvement of the vertebral arteries in giant cell arteritis mimicking vertebral dissection.**
  Author(s): Reinhard M, Schmidt D, Schumacher M, Hetzel A.
  Source: Journal of Neurology. 2003 August; 250(8): 1006-9. Erratum In: J Neurol. 2003 September; 250(9): 1134.
  http://www.ncbi.nlm.nih.gov/entrez/query.fcgi?cmd=Retrieve&db=pubmed&dopt=Abstract&list_uids=12928927

- **Is visual loss due to giant cell arteritis reversible?**
  Author(s): Calguneri M, Cobankara V, Ozatli D, Guler G, Apras S, Pay S, Kiraz S, Ertenli I, Ozturk MA.
  Source: Yonsei Medical Journal. 2003 February; 44(1): 155-8.
  http://www.ncbi.nlm.nih.gov/entrez/query.fcgi?cmd=Retrieve&db=pubmed&dopt=Abstract&list_uids=12619191

- **Isolated renal giant cell arteritis, not so rare a cause of renal failure?**
  Author(s): Scarpioni R, Poisetti PG, Cristinelli L, Zangrandi A.
  Source: American Journal of Kidney Diseases : the Official Journal of the National Kidney Foundation. 2003 March; 41(3): 720.
  http://www.ncbi.nlm.nih.gov/entrez/query.fcgi?cmd=Retrieve&db=pubmed&dopt=Abstract&list_uids=12613000

- **Isolated renal giant cell arteritis.**
  Author(s): Medvedev G, Al-Shamari AE, Copland MA, Magil AB.
  Source: American Journal of Kidney Diseases : the Official Journal of the National Kidney Foundation. 2002 September; 40(3): 658-61.
  http://www.ncbi.nlm.nih.gov/entrez/query.fcgi?cmd=Retrieve&db=pubmed&dopt=Abstract&list_uids=12200821

- **Laboratory investigations useful in giant cell arteritis and Takayasu's arteritis.**
  Author(s): Salvarani C, Cantini F, Boiardi L, Hunder GG.
  Source: Clin Exp Rheumatol. 2003 November-December; 21(6 Suppl 32): S23-8. Review.
  http://www.ncbi.nlm.nih.gov/entrez/query.fcgi?cmd=Retrieve&db=pubmed&dopt=Abstract&list_uids=14740424

- **Laboratory investigations useful in the evaluation of polymyalgia rheumatica (PMR) and giant cell arteritis (GCA).**
  Author(s): Hazleman B.
  Source: Clin Exp Rheumatol. 2000 July-August; 18(4 Suppl 20): S29-31. Review.
  http://www.ncbi.nlm.nih.gov/entrez/query.fcgi?cmd=Retrieve&db=pubmed&dopt=Abstract&list_uids=10948756

- **Lack of antineutrophil cytoplasmic antibodies as marker for giant cell arteritis.**
  Author(s): Nassberger L, Andersson R.
  Source: The Journal of Rheumatology. 1993 February; 20(2): 408-9.
  http://www.ncbi.nlm.nih.gov/entrez/query.fcgi?cmd=Retrieve&db=pubmed&dopt=Abstract&list_uids=8474095

- **Lack of association between altitude and incidence of giant cell arteritis in Northwest Spain.**
  Author(s): Llorca J, Bringas-Bollada M, Amor-Dorado JC, Garcia-Porrua C, Gonzalez-Gay MA.
  Source: Clin Exp Rheumatol. 2004 March-April; 22(2): 270. No Abstract Available.
  http://www.ncbi.nlm.nih.gov/entrez/query.fcgi?cmd=Retrieve&db=pubmed&dopt=Abstract&list_uids=15083905

- **Lack of association between IL-1 cluster and TNF-alpha gene polymorphisms and giant cell arteritis.**
  Author(s): Gonzalez-Gay MA, Di Giovine FS, Silvestri T, Amoli MM, Garcia-Porrua C, Thomson W, Ollier WE, Hajeer AH.
  Source: Clin Exp Rheumatol. 2002 May-June; 20(3): 431. No Abstract Available.
  http://www.ncbi.nlm.nih.gov/entrez/query.fcgi?cmd=Retrieve&db=pubmed&dopt=Abstract&list_uids=12102486

- **Lack of association between intercellular adhesion molecule-1 gene polymorphisms and giant cell arteritis.**
  Author(s): Amoli MM, Shelley E, Mattey DL, Garcia-Porrua C, Thomson W, Hajeer AH, Ollier WE, Gonzalez-Gay MA.
  Source: The Journal of Rheumatology. 2001 July; 28(7): 1600-4.
  http://www.ncbi.nlm.nih.gov/entrez/query.fcgi?cmd=Retrieve&db=pubmed&dopt=Abstract&list_uids=11469468

- **Lack of evidence for an association between hantavirus infections and Wegener's granulomatosis, microscopic polyangiitis, Churg-Strauss syndrome and giant cell arteritis.**
  Author(s): Gerke P, Wichmann D, Schonermarck U, Schutt M, Feldmann H, Ksiazek TG, Rob PM, Gross WL.
  Source: Rheumatology (Oxford, England). 2000 December; 39(12): 1424-5.
  http://www.ncbi.nlm.nih.gov/entrez/query.fcgi?cmd=Retrieve&db=pubmed&dopt=Abstract&list_uids=11136889

- **Large artery giant cell arteritis: a diagnosis to remember.**
  Author(s): Caramaschi P, Biasi D, Carletto A, Zeminian S, Manzo T, Bambara LM.
  Source: Clinical Rheumatology. 1997 March; 16(2): 219-20.
  http://www.ncbi.nlm.nih.gov/entrez/query.fcgi?cmd=Retrieve&db=pubmed&dopt=Abstract&list_uids=9093809

- **Large vessel vasculitis (giant cell arteritis, Takayasu arteritis).**
  Author(s): Wilke WS.
  Source: Baillieres Clin Rheumatol. 1997 May; 11(2): 285-313. Review.
  http://www.ncbi.nlm.nih.gov/entrez/query.fcgi?cmd=Retrieve&db=pubmed&dopt=Abstract&list_uids=9220079

- Large vessel vasculitis without temporal artery involvement: isolated form of giant cell arteritis?
  Author(s): Lambert M, Weber A, Boland B, De Plaen JF, Donckier J.
  Source: Clinical Rheumatology. 1996 March; 15(2): 174-80.
  http://www.ncbi.nlm.nih.gov/entrez/query.fcgi?cmd=Retrieve&db=pubmed&dopt=A bstract&list_uids=8777852

- Late ipsilateral recurrence of ischemic optic neuropathy in giant cell arteritis.
  Author(s): Kim N, Trobe JD, Flint A, Keoleian G.
  Source: Journal of Neuro-Ophthalmology : the Official Journal of the North American Neuro-Ophthalmology Society. 2003 June; 23(2): 122-6.
  http://www.ncbi.nlm.nih.gov/entrez/query.fcgi?cmd=Retrieve&db=pubmed&dopt=A bstract&list_uids=12782923

- Lipoprotein(a) and anticardiolipin antibodies as risk factors for thrombotic events in polymyalgia rheumatica and giant cell arteritis.
  Author(s): Seriolo B, Accardo S, Cutolo M.
  Source: The Journal of Rheumatology. 1996 August; 23(8): 1478-80.
  http://www.ncbi.nlm.nih.gov/entrez/query.fcgi?cmd=Retrieve&db=pubmed&dopt=A bstract&list_uids=8856634

- Liver involvement in giant cell arteritis.
  Author(s): Ilan Y, Ben-Chetrit E.
  Source: Clinical Rheumatology. 1993 June; 12(2): 219-22. Review.
  http://www.ncbi.nlm.nih.gov/entrez/query.fcgi?cmd=Retrieve&db=pubmed&dopt=A bstract&list_uids=8358982

- Longterm survival in acute rhinocerebral mucormycosis with giant cell arteritis and foreign body granulomas.
  Author(s): Castillo L, Hofman V, Betis F, Piche M, Roger PM, Santini J, Hofman P.
  Source: Pathology, Research and Practice. 2001; 197(3): 199-203.
  http://www.ncbi.nlm.nih.gov/entrez/query.fcgi?cmd=Retrieve&db=pubmed&dopt=A bstract&list_uids=11314785

- Long-term survival of patients with giant cell arteritis in the American College of Rheumatology giant cell arteritis classification criteria cohort.
  Author(s): Matteson EL, Gold KN, Bloch DA, Hunder GG.
  Source: The American Journal of Medicine. 1996 February; 100(2): 193-6.
  http://www.ncbi.nlm.nih.gov/entrez/query.fcgi?cmd=Retrieve&db=pubmed&dopt=A bstract&list_uids=8629654

- Low diagnostic yield with second biopsies in suspected giant cell arteritis.
  Author(s): Danesh-Meyer HV, Savino PJ, Eagle RC Jr, Kubis KC, Sergott RC.
  Source: Journal of Neuro-Ophthalmology : the Official Journal of the North American Neuro-Ophthalmology Society. 2000 September; 20(3): 213-5.
  http://www.ncbi.nlm.nih.gov/entrez/query.fcgi?cmd=Retrieve&db=pubmed&dopt=A bstract&list_uids=11001197

- **Low-dose aspirin and prevention of cranial ischemic complications in giant cell arteritis.**
  Author(s): Nesher G, Berkun Y, Mates M, Baras M, Rubinow A, Sonnenblick M.
  Source: Arthritis and Rheumatism. 2004 April; 50(4): 1332-7.
  http://www.ncbi.nlm.nih.gov/entrez/query.fcgi?cmd=Retrieve&db=pubmed&dopt=Abstract&list_uids=15077317

- **Low-dose aspirin in the treatment of giant cell arteritis.**
  Author(s): Hellmann DB.
  Source: Arthritis and Rheumatism. 2004 April; 50(4): 1026-7. Review.
  http://www.ncbi.nlm.nih.gov/entrez/query.fcgi?cmd=Retrieve&db=pubmed&dopt=Abstract&list_uids=15077284

- **Low-dose corticosteroids and blindness in giant cell arteritis.**
  Author(s): Gonzalez-Gay MA, Santiago J, Monte R, Blanco R.
  Source: British Journal of Rheumatology. 1996 July; 35(7): 702-3.
  http://www.ncbi.nlm.nih.gov/entrez/query.fcgi?cmd=Retrieve&db=pubmed&dopt=Abstract&list_uids=8758611

- **Lower limb giant cell arteritis and temporal arteritis: followup of 8 cases.**
  Author(s): Le Hello C, Levesque H, Jeanton M, Cailleux N, Galateau F, Peillon C, Veyssier P, Watelet J, Letellier P, Courtois H, Maiza D.
  Source: The Journal of Rheumatology. 2001 June; 28(6): 1407-12.
  http://www.ncbi.nlm.nih.gov/entrez/query.fcgi?cmd=Retrieve&db=pubmed&dopt=Abstract&list_uids=11409140

- **Magnetic resonance angiography in the diagnosis of a case of giant cell arteritis manifesting as scalp necrosis.**
  Author(s): Botella-Estrada R, Sammartin O, Martinez V, Campos S, Aliaga A.
  Source: Archives of Dermatology. 1999 July; 135(7): 769-71.
  http://www.ncbi.nlm.nih.gov/entrez/query.fcgi?cmd=Retrieve&db=pubmed&dopt=Abstract&list_uids=10411150

- **Management of giant cell arteritis and polymyalgia rheumatica.**
  Author(s): Meskimen S, Cook TD, Blake RL Jr.
  Source: American Family Physician. 2000 April 1; 61(7): 2061-8, 2073. Review.
  http://www.ncbi.nlm.nih.gov/entrez/query.fcgi?cmd=Retrieve&db=pubmed&dopt=Abstract&list_uids=10779249

- **Management of giant cell arteritis. Our 27-year clinical study: new light on old controversies.**
  Author(s): Hayreh SS, Zimmerman B.
  Source: Ophthalmologica. Journal International D'ophtalmologie. International Journal of Ophthalmology. Zeitschrift Fur Augenheilkunde. 2003 July-August; 217(4): 239-59.
  http://www.ncbi.nlm.nih.gov/entrez/query.fcgi?cmd=Retrieve&db=pubmed&dopt=Abstract&list_uids=12792130

- **Managing polymyalgia rheumatica and giant cell arteritis in the primary care setting.**
  Author(s): Terrazas D, Schumann L.
  Source: Journal of the American Academy of Nurse Practitioners. 1997 June; 9(6): 289-92, Quiz 294-6.
  http://www.ncbi.nlm.nih.gov/entrez/query.fcgi?cmd=Retrieve&db=pubmed&dopt=Abstract&list_uids=9274251

- **Mannose-binding lectin variant alleles and HLA-DR4 alleles are associated with giant cell arteritis.**
  Author(s): Jacobsen S, Baslund B, Madsen HO, Tvede N, Svejgaard A, Garred P.
  Source: The Journal of Rheumatology. 2002 October; 29(10): 2148-53.
  http://www.ncbi.nlm.nih.gov/entrez/query.fcgi?cmd=Retrieve&db=pubmed&dopt=Abstract&list_uids=12375325

- **Masticatory muscle pain: an important indicator of giant cell arteritis.**
  Author(s): Hayreh SS.
  Source: Spec Care Dentist. 1998 March-April; 18(2): 60-5.
  http://www.ncbi.nlm.nih.gov/entrez/query.fcgi?cmd=Retrieve&db=pubmed&dopt=Abstract&list_uids=9680912

- **Matrix metalloproteinases and tissue inhibitors of metalloproteinases in giant cell arteritis: an immunocytochemical study.**
  Author(s): Tomita T, Imakawa K.
  Source: Pathology. 1998 February; 30(1): 40-50.
  http://www.ncbi.nlm.nih.gov/entrez/query.fcgi?cmd=Retrieve&db=pubmed&dopt=Abstract&list_uids=9534207

- **Meniere's syndrome: an atypical presentation of giant cell arteritis (temporal arteritis).**
  Author(s): McKennan KX, Nielsen SL, Watson C, Wiesner K.
  Source: The Laryngoscope. 1993 October; 103(10): 1103-7.
  http://www.ncbi.nlm.nih.gov/entrez/query.fcgi?cmd=Retrieve&db=pubmed&dopt=Abstract&list_uids=8412445

- **Meningoradiculitis associated with giant cell arteritis.**
  Author(s): Roelcke U, Eschle D, Kappos L, Moschopulos M, Laeng RH, Buettner UW.
  Source: Neurology. 2002 December 10; 59(11): 1811-2.
  http://www.ncbi.nlm.nih.gov/entrez/query.fcgi?cmd=Retrieve&db=pubmed&dopt=Abstract&list_uids=12473783

- **Methotrexate treatment in the management of giant cell arteritis.**
  Author(s): Hernandez-Garcia C, Soriano C, Morado C, Ramos P, Fernandez-Gutierrez B, Herrero M, Banares A, Jover JA.
  Source: Scandinavian Journal of Rheumatology. 1994; 23(6): 295-8.
  http://www.ncbi.nlm.nih.gov/entrez/query.fcgi?cmd=Retrieve&db=pubmed&dopt=Abstract&list_uids=7801052

- **Microscopic haematuria in giant cell arteritis.**
  Author(s): Vanderschueren S, Depoot I, Knockaert DC, Verbeken EK, Zaman Z, Bobbaers H.
  Source: Clinical Rheumatology. 2002 September; 21(5): 373-7.
  http://www.ncbi.nlm.nih.gov/entrez/query.fcgi?cmd=Retrieve&db=pubmed&dopt=Abstract&list_uids=12223984

- **Molecular approaches toward pathologic mechanisms in giant cell arteritis and Takayasu's arteritis.**
  Author(s): Weyand CM, Goronzy JJ.
  Source: Current Opinion in Rheumatology. 1995 January; 7(1): 30-6. Review.
  http://www.ncbi.nlm.nih.gov/entrez/query.fcgi?cmd=Retrieve&db=pubmed&dopt=Abstract&list_uids=7718419

- **Morphological aspects of giant cells in giant cell arteritis: an electron-microscopic and immunocytochemical study.**
  Author(s): Nordborg E, Bengtsson BA, Petursdottir V, Nordborg C.
  Source: Clin Exp Rheumatol. 1997 March-April; 15(2): 129-34.
  http://www.ncbi.nlm.nih.gov/entrez/query.fcgi?cmd=Retrieve&db=pubmed&dopt=Abstract&list_uids=9196863

- **Mortality of large-artery complication (aortic aneurysm, aortic dissection, and/or large-artery stenosis) in patients with giant cell arteritis: a population-based study over 50 years.**
  Author(s): Nuenninghoff DM, Hunder GG, Christianson TJ, McClelland RL, Matteson EL.
  Source: Arthritis and Rheumatism. 2003 December; 48(12): 3532-7.
  http://www.ncbi.nlm.nih.gov/entrez/query.fcgi?cmd=Retrieve&db=pubmed&dopt=Abstract&list_uids=14674005

- **Multiple cerebral abscesses in a woman with giant cell arteritis.**
  Author(s): Cantalejo-Moreira M, Villaverde-Garcia V, Villlalba-Yllan A, Martin-Mola E.
  Source: Clin Exp Rheumatol. 2000 March-April; 18(2): 267. No Abstract Available.
  http://www.ncbi.nlm.nih.gov/entrez/query.fcgi?cmd=Retrieve&db=pubmed&dopt=Abstract&list_uids=10812509

- **Multiple myeloma-associated amyloidosis and giant cell arteritis.**
  Author(s): Estrada A, Stenzel TT, Burchette JL, Allen NB.
  Source: Arthritis and Rheumatism. 1998 July; 41(7): 1312-7.
  http://www.ncbi.nlm.nih.gov/entrez/query.fcgi?cmd=Retrieve&db=pubmed&dopt=Abstract&list_uids=9663490

- **Multiple strokes after initiation of steroid therapy in giant cell arteritis.**
  Author(s): Collazos J, Garcia-Monco C, Martin A, Rodriguez J, Gomez MA.
  Source: Postgraduate Medical Journal. 1994 March; 70(821): 228-30.
  http://www.ncbi.nlm.nih.gov/entrez/query.fcgi?cmd=Retrieve&db=pubmed&dopt=Abstract&list_uids=8183760

- Musculoskeletal manifestations in a population-based cohort of patients with giant cell arteritis.
  Author(s): Salvarani C, Hunder GG.
  Source: Arthritis and Rheumatism. 1999 June; 42(6): 1259-66.
  http://www.ncbi.nlm.nih.gov/entrez/query.fcgi?cmd=Retrieve&db=pubmed&dopt=Abstract&list_uids=10366120

- Myelodysplastic and myeloproliferative syndromes associated with giant cell arteritis and polymyalgia rheumatica: a coincidental coexistence or a causal relationship?
  Author(s): Espinosa G, Font J, Munoz-Rodriguez FJ, Cervera R, Ingelmo M.
  Source: Clinical Rheumatology. 2002 August; 21(4): 309-13.
  http://www.ncbi.nlm.nih.gov/entrez/query.fcgi?cmd=Retrieve&db=pubmed&dopt=Abstract&list_uids=12189460

- Myocardial infarction and coronary artery involvement in giant cell arteritis.
  Author(s): Freddo T, Price M, Kase C, Goldstein MP.
  Source: Optometry and Vision Science : Official Publication of the American Academy of Optometry. 1999 January; 76(1): 14-8.
  http://www.ncbi.nlm.nih.gov/entrez/query.fcgi?cmd=Retrieve&db=pubmed&dopt=Abstract&list_uids=10030611

- Necrosis of the lip in giant cell arteritis: report of a case.
  Author(s): Scully C, Eveson JW, Barrett AW, Cunningham SJ.
  Source: Journal of Oral and Maxillofacial Surgery : Official Journal of the American Association of Oral and Maxillofacial Surgeons. 1993 May; 51(5): 581-3. Review.
  http://www.ncbi.nlm.nih.gov/entrez/query.fcgi?cmd=Retrieve&db=pubmed&dopt=Abstract&list_uids=8478767

- Neovascularization around the optic nerve in giant cell arteritis.
  Author(s): Garcia-Porrua C, Pego-Reigosa R, Armesto V, Gonzalez-Gay MA.
  Source: Arthritis and Rheumatism. 2003 October 15; 49(5): 737-8.
  http://www.ncbi.nlm.nih.gov/entrez/query.fcgi?cmd=Retrieve&db=pubmed&dopt=Abstract&list_uids=14558066

- Neurologic manifestations of giant cell arteritis.
  Author(s): Nesher G.
  Source: Clin Exp Rheumatol. 2000 July-August; 18(4 Suppl 20): S24-6. Review.
  http://www.ncbi.nlm.nih.gov/entrez/query.fcgi?cmd=Retrieve&db=pubmed&dopt=Abstract&list_uids=10948754

- Neurologic manifestations of giant cell arteritis.
  Author(s): Reich KA, Giansiracusa DF, Strongwater SL.
  Source: The American Journal of Medicine. 1990 July; 89(1): 67-72. Review.
  http://www.ncbi.nlm.nih.gov/entrez/query.fcgi?cmd=Retrieve&db=pubmed&dopt=Abstract&list_uids=2195891

- **Neuro-ophthalmic complications of biopsy-proven giant cell arteritis.**
  Author(s): Glutz von Blotzheim S, Borruat FX.
  Source: Eur J Ophthalmol. 1997 October-December; 7(4): 375-82.
  http://www.ncbi.nlm.nih.gov/entrez/query.fcgi?cmd=Retrieve&db=pubmed&dopt=A
  bstract&list_uids=9457462

- **No additive effect of cyclosporin A compared with glucocorticoid treatment alone in giant cell arteritis: results of an open, controlled, randomized study.**
  Author(s): Schaufelberger C, Andersson R, Nordborg E.
  Source: British Journal of Rheumatology. 1998 April; 37(4): 464-5.
  http://www.ncbi.nlm.nih.gov/entrez/query.fcgi?cmd=Retrieve&db=pubmed&dopt=A
  bstract&list_uids=9619904

- **No evidence of parvovirus B19, Chlamydia pneumoniae or human herpes virus infection in temporal artery biopsies in patients with giant cell arteritis.**
  Author(s): Helweg-Larsen J, Tarp B, Obel N, Baslund B.
  Source: Rheumatology (Oxford, England). 2002 April; 41(4): 445-9.
  http://www.ncbi.nlm.nih.gov/entrez/query.fcgi?cmd=Retrieve&db=pubmed&dopt=A
  bstract&list_uids=11961176

- **Normal sedimentation rates and giant cell arteritis.**
  Author(s): Litwin MS, Henderson DR, Kirkham B.
  Source: Archives of Internal Medicine. 1992 January; 152(1): 209.
  http://www.ncbi.nlm.nih.gov/entrez/query.fcgi?cmd=Retrieve&db=pubmed&dopt=A
  bstract&list_uids=1728919

- **Occipital headache as a manifestation of giant cell arteritis.**
  Author(s): Blaiss MS, Waxman J, Lange RK.
  Source: Southern Medical Journal. 1982 July; 75(7): 887-8.
  http://www.ncbi.nlm.nih.gov/entrez/query.fcgi?cmd=Retrieve&db=pubmed&dopt=A
  bstract&list_uids=7089662

- **Occult giant cell arteritis: ocular manifestations.**
  Author(s): Hayreh SS, Podhajsky PA, Zimmerman B.
  Source: American Journal of Ophthalmology. 1998 April; 125(4): 521-6. Erratum In: Am J Ophthalmol 1998 June; 125(6): 893.
  http://www.ncbi.nlm.nih.gov/entrez/query.fcgi?cmd=Retrieve&db=pubmed&dopt=A
  bstract&list_uids=9559738

- **Ocular involvements of Japanese patients with giant cell arteritis from the first nation-wide survey.**
  Author(s): Kobayashi S, Yano T, Inaba Y, Hashimoto H, Matsumoto Y, Tamakoshi A, Kawamura T, Ohno Y.
  Source: Arthritis and Rheumatism. 2003 December 15; 49(6): 867-8.
  http://www.ncbi.nlm.nih.gov/entrez/query.fcgi?cmd=Retrieve&db=pubmed&dopt=A
  bstract&list_uids=14673978

- **Ocular manifestations of giant cell arteritis.**
  Author(s): Tovilla-Canales JL.
  Source: Current Opinion in Ophthalmology. 1998 December; 9(6): 73-9. Review.
  http://www.ncbi.nlm.nih.gov/entrez/query.fcgi?cmd=Retrieve&db=pubmed&dopt=Abstract&list_uids=10387340

- **Ocular manifestations of giant cell arteritis.**
  Author(s): Lee AG.
  Source: American Journal of Ophthalmology. 1998 November; 126(5): 742-4.
  http://www.ncbi.nlm.nih.gov/entrez/query.fcgi?cmd=Retrieve&db=pubmed&dopt=Abstract&list_uids=9822250

- **Ocular manifestations of giant cell arteritis.**
  Author(s): Hayreh SS, Podhajsky PA, Zimmerman B.
  Source: American Journal of Ophthalmology. 1998 April; 125(4): 509-20.
  http://www.ncbi.nlm.nih.gov/entrez/query.fcgi?cmd=Retrieve&db=pubmed&dopt=Abstract&list_uids=9559737

- **One hundred transient monocular central retinal artery occlusions secondary to giant cell arteritis.**
  Author(s): Alwitry A, Holden R.
  Source: Archives of Ophthalmology. 2003 December; 121(12): 1802-3.
  http://www.ncbi.nlm.nih.gov/entrez/query.fcgi?cmd=Retrieve&db=pubmed&dopt=Abstract&list_uids=14662610

- **Ophthalmic artery microembolism in giant cell arteritis.**
  Author(s): Schauble B, Wijman CA, Koleini B, Babikian VL.
  Source: Journal of Neuro-Ophthalmology : the Official Journal of the North American Neuro-Ophthalmology Society. 2000 December; 20(4): 273-5.
  http://www.ncbi.nlm.nih.gov/entrez/query.fcgi?cmd=Retrieve&db=pubmed&dopt=Abstract&list_uids=11130757

- **Oral and intravenous steroids in giant cell arteritis.**
  Author(s): Chan CC, O'Day J.
  Source: Clinical & Experimental Ophthalmology. 2003 June; 31(3): 179-82. Review.
  http://www.ncbi.nlm.nih.gov/entrez/query.fcgi?cmd=Retrieve&db=pubmed&dopt=Abstract&list_uids=12786766

- **Oral necrosis accompanying giant cell arteritis.**
  Author(s): Browne WG.
  Source: Journal of Oral and Maxillofacial Surgery : Official Journal of the American Association of Oral and Maxillofacial Surgeons. 1982 July; 40(7): 450-3.
  http://www.ncbi.nlm.nih.gov/entrez/query.fcgi?cmd=Retrieve&db=pubmed&dopt=Abstract&list_uids=6953200

- **Orbital presentations of giant cell arteritis.**
  Author(s): Lee AG, Tang RA, Feldon SE, Pless M, Schiffman JS, Rubin RM, Rao N.
  Source: Graefe's Archive for Clinical and Experimental Ophthalmology = Albrecht Von Graefes Archiv Fur Klinische Und Experimentelle Ophthalmologie. 2001 July; 239(7): 509-13.
  http://www.ncbi.nlm.nih.gov/entrez/query.fcgi?cmd=Retrieve&db=pubmed&dopt=Abstract&list_uids=11521695

- **Pathogenic mechanisms in giant cell arteritis.**
  Author(s): Weyand CM, Goronzy JJ.
  Source: Cleve Clin J Med. 2002; 69 Suppl 2: Sii28-32. Review.
  http://www.ncbi.nlm.nih.gov/entrez/query.fcgi?cmd=Retrieve&db=pubmed&dopt=Abstract&list_uids=12086261

- **Pathogenic principles in giant cell arteritis.**
  Author(s): Weyand CM, Goronzy JJ.
  Source: International Journal of Cardiology. 2000 August 31; 75 Suppl 1: S9-S15; Discussion S17-9. Review.
  http://www.ncbi.nlm.nih.gov/entrez/query.fcgi?cmd=Retrieve&db=pubmed&dopt=Abstract&list_uids=10980331

- **Pericardial and pleural effusion in giant cell arteritis.**
  Author(s): Valstar MH, Terpstra WF, de Jong RS.
  Source: The American Journal of Medicine. 2003 June 1; 114(8): 708-9.
  http://www.ncbi.nlm.nih.gov/entrez/query.fcgi?cmd=Retrieve&db=pubmed&dopt=Abstract&list_uids=12798467

- **Polymyalgia rheumatica and biopsy-proven giant cell arteritis exhibit different HLA-DRB1* associations.**
  Author(s): Gonzalez-Gay MA, Garcia-Porrua C, Ollier WE.
  Source: The Journal of Rheumatology. 2003 December; 30(12): 2729.
  http://www.ncbi.nlm.nih.gov/entrez/query.fcgi?cmd=Retrieve&db=pubmed&dopt=Abstract&list_uids=14719228

- **Polymyalgia rheumatica and giant cell arteritis.**
  Author(s): Zilko PJ.
  Source: The Medical Journal of Australia. 1996 October 21; 165(8): 438-42. Review.
  http://www.ncbi.nlm.nih.gov/entrez/query.fcgi?cmd=Retrieve&db=pubmed&dopt=Abstract&list_uids=8913247

- **Polymyalgia rheumatica and giant cell arteritis.**
  Author(s): Evans JM, Hunder GG.
  Source: Rheumatic Diseases Clinics of North America. 2000 August; 26(3): 493-515. Review.
  http://www.ncbi.nlm.nih.gov/entrez/query.fcgi?cmd=Retrieve&db=pubmed&dopt=Abstract&list_uids=10989509

- Polymyalgia rheumatica and giant cell arteritis. Avoiding management traps.
  Author(s): de Jager JP.
  Source: Aust Fam Physician. 2001 July; 30(7): 643-7.
  http://www.ncbi.nlm.nih.gov/entrez/query.fcgi?cmd=Retrieve&db=pubmed&dopt=Abstract&list_uids=11558196

- Prognostic factors and long-term evolution in a cohort of 133 patients with giant cell arteritis.
  Author(s): Hachulla E, Boivin V, Pasturel-Michon U, Fauchais AL, Bouroz-Joly J, Perez-Cousin M, Hatron PY, Devulder B.
  Source: Clin Exp Rheumatol. 2001 March-April; 19(2): 171-6.
  http://www.ncbi.nlm.nih.gov/entrez/query.fcgi?cmd=Retrieve&db=pubmed&dopt=Abstract&list_uids=11326479

- Progressive visual loss from giant cell arteritis despite high-dose intravenous methylprednisolone.
  Author(s): Cornblath WT, Eggenberger ER.
  Source: Ophthalmology. 1997 May; 104(5): 854-8. Review.
  http://www.ncbi.nlm.nih.gov/entrez/query.fcgi?cmd=Retrieve&db=pubmed&dopt=Abstract&list_uids=9160034

- Pulmonary thromboendarterectomy in a patient with giant cell arteritis.
  Author(s): Brister SJ, Wilson-Yang K, Lobo FV, Yang H, Skala R.
  Source: The Annals of Thoracic Surgery. 2002 June; 73(6): 1977-9.
  http://www.ncbi.nlm.nih.gov/entrez/query.fcgi?cmd=Retrieve&db=pubmed&dopt=Abstract&list_uids=12078812

- Reactive nitrogen intermediates in giant cell arteritis: selective nitration of neocapillaries.
  Author(s): Borkowski A, Younge BR, Szweda L, Mock B, Bjornsson J, Moeller K, Goronzy JJ, Weyand CM.
  Source: American Journal of Pathology. 2002 July; 161(1): 115-23.
  http://www.ncbi.nlm.nih.gov/entrez/query.fcgi?cmd=Retrieve&db=pubmed&dopt=Abstract&list_uids=12107096

- Reappraisal of the epidemiology of giant cell arteritis in Olmsted County, Minnesota, over a fifty-year period.
  Author(s): Salvarani C, Crowson CS, O'Fallon WM, Hunder GG, Gabriel SE.
  Source: Arthritis and Rheumatism. 2004 April 15; 51(2): 264-8.
  http://www.ncbi.nlm.nih.gov/entrez/query.fcgi?cmd=Retrieve&db=pubmed&dopt=Abstract&list_uids=15077270

- Recognition of tissue residing antigen by T cells in vasculitic lesions of giant cell arteritis.
  Author(s): Martinez-Taboada V, Hunder NN, Hunder GG, Weyand CM, Goronzy JJ.
  Source: Journal of Molecular Medicine (Berlin, Germany). 1996 November; 74(11): 695-703.
  http://www.ncbi.nlm.nih.gov/entrez/query.fcgi?cmd=Retrieve&db=pubmed&dopt=Abstract&list_uids=8956156

- **Recovery of visual function in patients with biopsy-proven giant cell arteritis.**
  Author(s): Foroozan R, Deramo VA, Buono LM, Jayamanne DG, Sergott RC, Danesh-Meyer H, Savino PJ.
  Source: Ophthalmology. 2003 March; 110(3): 539-42. Review.
  http://www.ncbi.nlm.nih.gov/entrez/query.fcgi?cmd=Retrieve&db=pubmed&dopt=Abstract&list_uids=12623817

- **Reduction of jaw opening (trismus) in giant cell arteritis.**
  Author(s): Nir-Paz R, Gross A, Chajek-Shaul T.
  Source: Annals of the Rheumatic Diseases. 2002 September; 61(9): 832-3. Review.
  http://www.ncbi.nlm.nih.gov/entrez/query.fcgi?cmd=Retrieve&db=pubmed&dopt=Abstract&list_uids=12176811

- **Reduction of jaw opening in giant cell arteritis.**
  Author(s): Liozon E, Jauberteau MO, Ly K, Loustaud V, Soria P, Vidal E.
  Source: Annals of the Rheumatic Diseases. 2003 March; 62(3): 287-8; Author Reply 288.
  http://www.ncbi.nlm.nih.gov/entrez/query.fcgi?cmd=Retrieve&db=pubmed&dopt=Abstract&list_uids=12594132

- **Risk factors and predictive models of giant cell arteritis in polymyalgia rheumatica.**
  Author(s): Rodriguez-Valverde V, Sarabia JM, Gonzalez-Gay MA, Figueroa M, Armona J, Blanco R, Fernandez-Sueiro JL, Martinez-Taboada VM.
  Source: The American Journal of Medicine. 1997 April; 102(4): 331-6.
  http://www.ncbi.nlm.nih.gov/entrez/query.fcgi?cmd=Retrieve&db=pubmed&dopt=Abstract&list_uids=9217613

- **Risk factors for cranial ischemic complications in giant cell arteritis.**
  Author(s): Nesher G, Berkun Y, Mates M, Baras M, Nesher R, Rubinow A, Sonnenblick M.
  Source: Medicine; Analytical Reviews of General Medicine, Neurology, Psychiatry, Dermatology, and Pediatrics. 2004 March; 83(2): 114-22. Review.
  http://www.ncbi.nlm.nih.gov/entrez/query.fcgi?cmd=Retrieve&db=pubmed&dopt=Abstract&list_uids=15028965

- **Role for vascular investigations in giant cell arteritis.**
  Author(s): Ann Intern Med. 2002 Aug 20;137(4):I26
  Source: Joint, Bone, Spine : Revue Du Rhumatisme. 2002 June; 69(4): 367-72. Review.
  http://www.ncbi.nlm.nih.gov/entrez/query.fcgi?cmd=Retrieve&db=pubmed&dopt=Abstract&list_uids=12186537

- **Role of thrombocytosis in diagnosis of giant cell arteritis and differentiation of arteritic from non-arteritic anterior ischemic optic neuropathy.**
  Author(s): Costello F, Zimmerman MB, Podhajsky PA, Hayreh SS.
  Source: Eur J Ophthalmol. 2004 May-June; 14(3): 245-57.
  http://www.ncbi.nlm.nih.gov/entrez/query.fcgi?cmd=Retrieve&db=pubmed&dopt=Abstract&list_uids=15206651

- **Scalp necrosis in giant cell arteritis and review of the literature.**
  Author(s): Currey J.
  Source: British Journal of Rheumatology. 1997 July; 36(7): 814-6. Review.
  http://www.ncbi.nlm.nih.gov/entrez/query.fcgi?cmd=Retrieve&db=pubmed&dopt=A
  bstract&list_uids=9255121

- **Scalp necrosis: an unusual presentation of giant cell arteritis.**
  Author(s): Paletta CE, Dehghan K, Campbell TC, Roth FS.
  Source: Plastic and Reconstructive Surgery. 2002 April 1; 109(4): 1474-5.
  http://www.ncbi.nlm.nih.gov/entrez/query.fcgi?cmd=Retrieve&db=pubmed&dopt=A
  bstract&list_uids=11965023

- **Selective T cell receptor decrease in peripheral blood T lymphocytes of patients with polymyalgia rheumatica and giant cell arteritis.**
  Author(s): Lopez-Hoyos M, Bartolome-Pacheco MJ, Blanco R, Rodriguez-Valverde V, Martinez-Taboada VM.
  Source: Annals of the Rheumatic Diseases. 2004 January; 63(1): 54-60.
  http://www.ncbi.nlm.nih.gov/entrez/query.fcgi?cmd=Retrieve&db=pubmed&dopt=A
  bstract&list_uids=14672892

- **Serum soluble CD23 levels in giant cell arteritis.**
  Author(s): Roblot P, Morel F, Lelievre E, Biais-Sauvetre MH, de Groote D, Preud'homme JL, Lecron JC.
  Source: Immunology Letters. 1996 October; 53(1): 41-4.
  http://www.ncbi.nlm.nih.gov/entrez/query.fcgi?cmd=Retrieve&db=pubmed&dopt=A
  bstract&list_uids=8946216

- **Sex differences in giant cell arteritis.**
  Author(s): Nuenninghoff DM, Hunder GG, Matteson EL.
  Source: The Journal of Rheumatology. 2003 May; 30(5): 1119; Author Reply 1119-20.
  http://www.ncbi.nlm.nih.gov/entrez/query.fcgi?cmd=Retrieve&db=pubmed&dopt=A
  bstract&list_uids=12734921

- **Sex differences in giant cell arteritis.**
  Author(s): Nir-Paz R, Gross A, Chajek-Shaul T.
  Source: The Journal of Rheumatology. 2002 June; 29(6): 1219-23.
  http://www.ncbi.nlm.nih.gov/entrez/query.fcgi?cmd=Retrieve&db=pubmed&dopt=A
  bstract&list_uids=12064839

- **Siegrist streaks in giant cell arteritis.**
  Author(s): Coupal DJ, Patel AD.
  Source: Journal of Neuro-Ophthalmology : the Official Journal of the North American Neuro-Ophthalmology Society. 2003 December; 23(4): 272-3.
  http://www.ncbi.nlm.nih.gov/entrez/query.fcgi?cmd=Retrieve&db=pubmed&dopt=A
  bstract&list_uids=14663308

- **Silent, or masked, giant cell arteritis is associated with a strong inflammatory response and a benign short term course.**
  Author(s): Liozon E, Boutros-Toni F, Ly K, Loustaud-Ratti V, Soria P, Vidal E.
  Source: The Journal of Rheumatology. 2003 June; 30(6): 1272-6.
  http://www.ncbi.nlm.nih.gov/entrez/query.fcgi?cmd=Retrieve&db=pubmed&dopt=A bstract&list_uids=12784402

- **Simultaneous presentation of giant cell arteritis and chronic lymphocytic leukemia.**
  Author(s): Gonzalez-Gay MA, Blanco R, Gonzalez-Lopez MA.
  Source: The Journal of Rheumatology. 1997 February; 24(2): 407-8.
  http://www.ncbi.nlm.nih.gov/entrez/query.fcgi?cmd=Retrieve&db=pubmed&dopt=A bstract&list_uids=9035008

- **Successful treatment of resistant giant cell arteritis with etanercept.**
  Author(s): Tan AL, Holdsworth J, Pease C, Emery P, McGonagle D.
  Source: Annals of the Rheumatic Diseases. 2003 April; 62(4): 373-4.
  http://www.ncbi.nlm.nih.gov/entrez/query.fcgi?cmd=Retrieve&db=pubmed&dopt=A bstract&list_uids=12634246

- **Temporal artery biopsy diagnosis of giant cell arteritis: lessons from 1109 biopsies.**
  Author(s): Lie JT.
  Source: Anat Pathol. 1996; 1: 69-97. Review. No Abstract Available.
  http://www.ncbi.nlm.nih.gov/entrez/query.fcgi?cmd=Retrieve&db=pubmed&dopt=A bstract&list_uids=9390924

- **The epidemiology of biopsy-positive giant cell arteritis: special reference to changes in the age of the population.**
  Author(s): Nordborg C, Johansson H, Petursdottir V, Nordborg E.
  Source: Rheumatology (Oxford, England). 2003 April; 42(4): 549-52.
  http://www.ncbi.nlm.nih.gov/entrez/query.fcgi?cmd=Retrieve&db=pubmed&dopt=A bstract&list_uids=12649402

- **The implications of recognizing large-vessel involvement in elderly patients with giant cell arteritis.**
  Author(s): Evans J, Hunder GG.
  Source: Current Opinion in Rheumatology. 1997 January; 9(1): 37-40. Review.
  http://www.ncbi.nlm.nih.gov/entrez/query.fcgi?cmd=Retrieve&db=pubmed&dopt=A bstract&list_uids=9110132

- **The right place of 18FDG PET for the diagnosis of giant cell arteritis--a response to the article of Brodmann et al.**
  Author(s): Belhocine T.
  Source: Rheumatology (Oxford, England). 2004 May; 43(5): 675-6; Author Reply 676.
  http://www.ncbi.nlm.nih.gov/entrez/query.fcgi?cmd=Retrieve&db=pubmed&dopt=A bstract&list_uids=15103035

- **The role of 2-18F-fluoro-2-deoxy-D-glucose positron emission tomography in the diagnosis of giant cell arteritis of the temporal arteries.**
  Author(s): Brodmann M, Lipp RW, Passath A, Seinost G, Pabst E, Pilger E.
  Source: Rheumatology (Oxford, England). 2004 February; 43(2): 241-2. Epub 2003 September 16.
  http://www.ncbi.nlm.nih.gov/entrez/query.fcgi?cmd=Retrieve&db=pubmed&dopt=Abstract&list_uids=13130153

- **The use of ultrasound as an aid in the diagnosis of giant cell arteritis: a pilot study comparing histological features with ultrasound findings.**
  Author(s): Murgatroyd H, Nimmo M, Evans A, MacEwen C.
  Source: Eye (London, England). 2003 April; 17(3): 415-9.
  http://www.ncbi.nlm.nih.gov/entrez/query.fcgi?cmd=Retrieve&db=pubmed&dopt=Abstract&list_uids=12724706

- **Three year follow-up of a case of giant cell arteritis presenting with a chronic cough and upper limb ischaemic symptoms.**
  Author(s): Jolobe OM.
  Source: British Journal of Rheumatology. 1997 April; 36(4): 503.
  http://www.ncbi.nlm.nih.gov/entrez/query.fcgi?cmd=Retrieve&db=pubmed&dopt=Abstract&list_uids=9159551

- **Three year follow-up of a case of giant cell arteritis presenting with a chronic cough and upper limb ischaemic symptoms.**
  Author(s): Rischmueller M, Davies RP, Smith MD.
  Source: British Journal of Rheumatology. 1996 August; 35(8): 800-2.
  http://www.ncbi.nlm.nih.gov/entrez/query.fcgi?cmd=Retrieve&db=pubmed&dopt=Abstract&list_uids=8761197

- **Treatment of resistant giant cell arteritis with etanercept.**
  Author(s): Docken WP.
  Source: Annals of the Rheumatic Diseases. 2004 April; 63(4): 469; Author Reply 469-70.
  http://www.ncbi.nlm.nih.gov/entrez/query.fcgi?cmd=Retrieve&db=pubmed&dopt=Abstract&list_uids=15020354

- **Ulceration and necrosis of the tongue due to giant cell arteritis.**
  Author(s): Christensen L.
  Source: Acta Med Scand. 1986; 220(4): 379-80.
  http://www.ncbi.nlm.nih.gov/entrez/query.fcgi?cmd=Retrieve&db=pubmed&dopt=Abstract&list_uids=3799243

- **Ulcerative colitis and giant cell arteritis associated with sensorineural deafness.**
  Author(s): Jacob A, Ledingham JG, Kerr AI, Ford MJ.
  Source: The Journal of Laryngology and Otology. 1990 November; 104(11): 889-90.
  http://www.ncbi.nlm.nih.gov/entrez/query.fcgi?cmd=Retrieve&db=pubmed&dopt=Abstract&list_uids=2266315

- **Unilateral central retinal artery occlusion followed by contralateral anterior ischemic optic neuropathy in giant cell arteritis.**
  Author(s): Wein FB, Miller NR.
  Source: Retina (Philadelphia, Pa.). 2000; 20(3): 301-3.
  http://www.ncbi.nlm.nih.gov/entrez/query.fcgi?cmd=Retrieve&db=pubmed&dopt=Abstract&list_uids=10872938

- **Unilateral distal extremity swelling with pitting oedema in giant cell arteritis.**
  Author(s): Kontoyianni A, Maragou M, Alvanou E, Kappou I, Dantis P.
  Source: Clinical Rheumatology. 1999; 18(1): 82-4.
  http://www.ncbi.nlm.nih.gov/entrez/query.fcgi?cmd=Retrieve&db=pubmed&dopt=Abstract&list_uids=10088960

- **Unilateral painful shoulder: a very unusual presenting form of giant cell arteritis.**
  Author(s): Cid MC, Coca A, Campa MT, Vicens A.
  Source: The Journal of Rheumatology. 1988 August; 15(8): 1312-3.
  http://www.ncbi.nlm.nih.gov/entrez/query.fcgi?cmd=Retrieve&db=pubmed&dopt=Abstract&list_uids=3184081

- **Unsuspected giant cell arteritis diagnosed at open heart surgery.**
  Author(s): Kay RH, Pooley R, Herman MV.
  Source: Archives of Internal Medicine. 1982 July; 142(7): 1378-9.
  http://www.ncbi.nlm.nih.gov/entrez/query.fcgi?cmd=Retrieve&db=pubmed&dopt=Abstract&list_uids=6979987

- **Unusual manifestations of giant cell arteritis: pulmonary nodules, cough, conjunctivitis and otitis with deafness.**
  Author(s): Zenone T, Souquet PJ, Bohas C, Vital Durand D, Bernard JP.
  Source: The European Respiratory Journal : Official Journal of the European Society for Clinical Respiratory Physiology. 1994 December; 7(12): 2252-4.
  http://www.ncbi.nlm.nih.gov/entrez/query.fcgi?cmd=Retrieve&db=pubmed&dopt=Abstract&list_uids=7713213

- **Update on giant cell arteritis.**
  Author(s): Su GW, Foroozan R.
  Source: Current Opinion in Ophthalmology. 2003 December; 14(6): 332-8. Review.
  http://www.ncbi.nlm.nih.gov/entrez/query.fcgi?cmd=Retrieve&db=pubmed&dopt=Abstract&list_uids=14615636

- **Upper extremity vaso-occlusive disease in a patient with giant cell arteritis.**
  Author(s): Neuzil KM, Morgan HJ.
  Source: J Tenn Med Assoc. 1991 July; 84(7): 331-2. No Abstract Available.
  http://www.ncbi.nlm.nih.gov/entrez/query.fcgi?cmd=Retrieve&db=pubmed&dopt=Abstract&list_uids=1870346

- **Vascular endothelial growth factor gene polymorphisms in giant cell arteritis.**
  Author(s): Boiardi L, Casali B, Nicoli D, Farnetti E, Chen Q, Macchioni P, Catanoso MG, Pulsatelli L, Meliconi R, Salvarani C.
  Source: The Journal of Rheumatology. 2003 October; 30(10): 2160-4.
  http://www.ncbi.nlm.nih.gov/entrez/query.fcgi?cmd=Retrieve&db=pubmed&dopt=Abstract&list_uids=14528511

- **Vessel wall morphometry in giant cell arteritis.**
  Author(s): Nordborg C, Petursdottir V.
  Source: Arthritis Care and Research : the Official Journal of the Arthritis Health Professions Association. 2000 October; 13(5): 286-90.
  http://www.ncbi.nlm.nih.gov/entrez/query.fcgi?cmd=Retrieve&db=pubmed&dopt=Abstract&list_uids=14635297

- **Vision loss in giant cell arteritis patients treated with alternate-day corticosteroids: comment on the article by Hoffman et al.**
  Author(s): Spiera RF, Kupersmith M, Paget S, Spiera H.
  Source: Arthritis and Rheumatism. 2003 April; 48(4): 1159-60; Author Reply 1160-1.
  http://www.ncbi.nlm.nih.gov/entrez/query.fcgi?cmd=Retrieve&db=pubmed&dopt=Abstract&list_uids=12687562

- **Visual deterioration in giant cell arteritis patients while on high doses of corticosteroid therapy.**
  Author(s): Hayreh SS, Zimmerman B.
  Source: Ophthalmology. 2003 June; 110(6): 1204-15. Review.
  http://www.ncbi.nlm.nih.gov/entrez/query.fcgi?cmd=Retrieve&db=pubmed&dopt=Abstract&list_uids=12799248

- **Visual hallucinations in giant cell arteritis: association with visual loss.**
  Author(s): Nesher G, Nesher R, Rozenman Y, Sonnenblick M.
  Source: The Journal of Rheumatology. 2001 September; 28(9): 2046-8.
  http://www.ncbi.nlm.nih.gov/entrez/query.fcgi?cmd=Retrieve&db=pubmed&dopt=Abstract&list_uids=11550973

- **Visual improvement with corticosteroid therapy in giant cell arteritis. Report of a large study and review of literature.**
  Author(s): Hayreh SS, Zimmerman B, Kardon RH.
  Source: Acta Ophthalmologica Scandinavica. 2002 August; 80(4): 355-67. Review. Erratum In: Acta Ophthalmol Scand. 2002 December; 80(6): 688.
  http://www.ncbi.nlm.nih.gov/entrez/query.fcgi?cmd=Retrieve&db=pubmed&dopt=Abstract&list_uids=12190776

- **Visual loss and giant cell arteritis.**
  Author(s): Docken WP.
  Source: British Journal of Rheumatology. 1997 July; 36(7): 823.
  http://www.ncbi.nlm.nih.gov/entrez/query.fcgi?cmd=Retrieve&db=pubmed&dopt=Abstract&list_uids=9255128

- **Visual loss as the presenting feature of giant cell arteritis.**
  Author(s): Toh ML, Wicks IP.
  Source: Aust N Z J Med. 2000 December; 30(6): 734. No Abstract Available.
  http://www.ncbi.nlm.nih.gov/entrez/query.fcgi?cmd=Retrieve&db=pubmed&dopt=Abstract&list_uids=11198589

- **Visual recovery after retinal stroke due to giant cell arteritis.**
  Author(s): Barbazan C, Gonzalez-Gay MA, Aspe B, Fucinos L, Mantecon-Aparicio JM.
  Source: Clin Exp Rheumatol. 2000 May-June; 18(3): 425-6. No Abstract Available.
  http://www.ncbi.nlm.nih.gov/entrez/query.fcgi?cmd=Retrieve&db=pubmed&dopt=Abstract&list_uids=10895393

- **Von Willebrand factor in polymyalgia rheumatica and giant cell arteritis.**
  Author(s): Uddhammar AC.
  Source: Clin Exp Rheumatol. 2000 July-August; 18(4 Suppl 20): S32-3. Review.
  http://www.ncbi.nlm.nih.gov/entrez/query.fcgi?cmd=Retrieve&db=pubmed&dopt=Abstract&list_uids=10948757

- **What is the appropriate initial dose of corticosteroids to treat giant cell arteritis?**
  Author(s): Wilke WS.
  Source: Cleve Clin J Med. 2000 August; 67(8): 546-8. No Abstract Available.
  http://www.ncbi.nlm.nih.gov/entrez/query.fcgi?cmd=Retrieve&db=pubmed&dopt=Abstract&list_uids=10946446

- **When to suspect giant cell arteritis.**
  Author(s): Healey LA.
  Source: Med Times. 1977 February; 105(2): 33D-35D. No Abstract Available.
  http://www.ncbi.nlm.nih.gov/entrez/query.fcgi?cmd=Retrieve&db=pubmed&dopt=Abstract&list_uids=834130

- **YKL-40 in giant cells and macrophages from patients with giant cell arteritis.**
  Author(s): Johansen JS, Baslund B, Garbarsch C, Hansen M, Stoltenberg M, Lorenzen I, Price PA.
  Source: Arthritis and Rheumatism. 1999 December; 42(12): 2624-30.
  http://www.ncbi.nlm.nih.gov/entrez/query.fcgi?cmd=Retrieve&db=pubmed&dopt=Abstract&list_uids=10616010

CHAPTER 2. NUTRITION AND GIANT CELL ARTERITIS

Overview

In this chapter, we will show you how to find studies dedicated specifically to nutrition and giant cell arteritis.

Finding Nutrition Studies on Giant Cell Arteritis

The National Institutes of Health's Office of Dietary Supplements (ODS) offers a searchable bibliographic database called the IBIDS (International Bibliographic Information on Dietary Supplements; National Institutes of Health, Building 31, Room 1B29, 31 Center Drive, MSC 2086, Bethesda, Maryland 20892-2086, Tel: 301-435-2920, Fax: 301-480-1845, E-mail: ods@nih.gov). The IBIDS contains over 460,000 scientific citations and summaries about dietary supplements and nutrition as well as references to published international, scientific literature on dietary supplements such as vitamins, minerals, and botanicals.[7] The IBIDS includes references and citations to both human and animal research studies.

As a service of the ODS, access to the IBIDS database is available free of charge at the following Web address: **http://ods.od.nih.gov/databases/ibids.html**. After entering the search area, you have three choices: (1) IBIDS Consumer Database, (2) Full IBIDS Database, or (3) Peer Reviewed Citations Only.

Now that you have selected a database, click on the "Advanced" tab. An advanced search allows you to retrieve up to 100 fully explained references in a comprehensive format. Type "giant cell arteritis" (or synonyms) into the search box, and click "Go." To narrow the search, you can also select the "Title" field.

---

[7] Adapted from **http://ods.od.nih.gov**. IBIDS is produced by the Office of Dietary Supplements (ODS) at the National Institutes of Health to assist the public, healthcare providers, educators, and researchers in locating credible, scientific information on dietary supplements. IBIDS was developed and will be maintained through an interagency partnership with the Food and Nutrition Information Center of the National Agricultural Library, U.S. Department of Agriculture.

The following information is typical of that found when using the "Full IBIDS Database" to search for "giant cell arteritis" (or a synonym):

- **Bone mineral density in patients with temporal arteritis and polymyalgia rheumatica.**
  Author(s): Rheumatology Service, Hospital de Bellvitge Princeps d'Espanya, Barcelona, Spain.
  Source: Mateo, L Nolla, J M Rozadilla, A Rodriguez Moreno, J Niubo, R Valverde, J Roig Escofet, D J-Rheumatol. 1993 August; 20(8): 1369-73 0315-162X

- **Prevalence and evolution of anticardiolipin antibodies in giant cell arteritis during corticosteroid therapy. A prospective study of 20 consecutive cases.**
  Author(s): Clinique Medicale, CHU Rouen, France.
  Source: Kerleau, J M Levesque, H Delpech, A Cailleux, N Chassagne, P Mejjad, O Manchon, N D Bercoff, E Tron, F Courtois, H et al. Br-J-Rheumatol. 1994 July; 33(7): 648-50 0263-7103

- **Visual performance in giant cell arteritis (temporal arteritis) after 1 year of therapy.**
  Author(s): INN at Beth Israel Medical Center, New York, NY 10128, USA.
  Source: Kupersmith, M J Langer, R Mitnick, H Spiera, R Spiera, H Richmond, M Paget, S Br-J-Ophthalmol. 1999 July; 83(7): 796-801 0007-1161

Federal Resources on Nutrition

In addition to the IBIDS, the United States Department of Health and Human Services (HHS) and the United States Department of Agriculture (USDA) provide many sources of information on general nutrition and health. Recommended resources include:

- healthfinder®, HHS's gateway to health information, including diet and nutrition: **http://www.healthfinder.gov/scripts/SearchContext.asp?topic=238&page=0**

- The United States Department of Agriculture's Web site dedicated to nutrition information: **www.nutrition.gov**

- The Food and Drug Administration's Web site for federal food safety information: **www.foodsafety.gov**

- The National Action Plan on Overweight and Obesity sponsored by the United States Surgeon General: **http://www.surgeongeneral.gov/topics/obesity/**

- The Center for Food Safety and Applied Nutrition has an Internet site sponsored by the Food and Drug Administration and the Department of Health and Human Services: **http://vm.cfsan.fda.gov/**

- Center for Nutrition Policy and Promotion sponsored by the United States Department of Agriculture: **http://www.usda.gov/cnpp/**

- Food and Nutrition Information Center, National Agricultural Library sponsored by the United States Department of Agriculture: **http://www.nal.usda.gov/fnic/**

- Food and Nutrition Service sponsored by the United States Department of Agriculture: **http://www.fns.usda.gov/fns/**

Additional Web Resources

A number of additional Web sites offer encyclopedic information covering food and nutrition. The following is a representative sample:

- AOL: **http://search.aol.com/cat.adp?id=174&layer=&from=subcats**

- Family Village: **http://www.familyvillage.wisc.edu/med_nutrition.html**

- Google: **http://directory.google.com/Top/Health/Nutrition/**

- Healthnotes: **http://www.healthnotes.com/**

- Open Directory Project: **http://dmoz.org/Health/Nutrition/**

- Yahoo.com: **http://dir.yahoo.com/Health/Nutrition/**

- WebMD®Health: **http://my.webmd.com/nutrition**

- WholeHealthMD.com: **http://www.wholehealthmd.com/reflib/0,1529,00.html**

CHAPTER 3. ALTERNATIVE MEDICINE AND GIANT CELL ARTERITIS

Overview

In this chapter, we will begin by introducing you to official information sources on complementary and alternative medicine (CAM) relating to giant cell arteritis. At the conclusion of this chapter, we will provide additional sources.

National Center for Complementary and Alternative Medicine

The National Center for Complementary and Alternative Medicine (NCCAM) of the National Institutes of Health (**http://nccam.nih.gov/**) has created a link to the National Library of Medicine's databases to facilitate research for articles that specifically relate to giant cell arteritis and complementary medicine. To search the database, go to the following Web site: **http://www.nlm.nih.gov/nccam/camonpubmed.html**. Select "CAM on PubMed." Enter "giant cell arteritis" (or synonyms) into the search box. Click "Go." The following references provide information on particular aspects of complementary and alternative medicine that are related to giant cell arteritis:

- **Anterior ischemic optic neuropathy.**
  Author(s): Hayreh SS.
  Source: Clin Neurosci. 1997; 4(5): 251-63. Review.
  http://www.ncbi.nlm.nih.gov/entrez/query.fcgi?cmd=Retrieve&db=pubmed&dopt=Abstract&list_uids=9292252

- **Anterior ischemic optic neuropathy: sense and nonsense in diagnosis and treatment.**
  Author(s): Bastiaensen LA, Keunen RW, Tijssen CC, Vandoninck JJ.
  Source: Documenta Ophthalmologica. Advances in Ophthalmology. 1986 January 15; 61(3-4): 205-10.
  http://www.ncbi.nlm.nih.gov/entrez/query.fcgi?cmd=Retrieve&db=pubmed&dopt=Abstract&list_uids=3512216

- **Auditory evoked phosphenes in optic nerve disease.**
  Author(s): Page NG, Bolger JP, Sanders MD.

Source: Journal of Neurology, Neurosurgery, and Psychiatry. 1982 January; 45(1): 7-12.
http://www.ncbi.nlm.nih.gov/entrez/query.fcgi?cmd=Retrieve&db=pubmed&dopt=Abstract&list_uids=7062073

- **Deflazacort in giant cell arteritis.**
  Author(s): Devogelaer JP, Gennari C.
  Source: The Journal of Rheumatology. 2002 October; 29(10): 2244-5.
  http://www.ncbi.nlm.nih.gov/entrez/query.fcgi?cmd=Retrieve&db=pubmed&dopt=Abstract&list_uids=12375347

- **Headache.**
  Author(s): Alden CB, Smith BH, Carson WR, Schumacher GA, Wallman LJ, Bissell GW, Boag TJ.
  Source: N Y State J Med. 1966 February 15; 66(4): 467-86. No Abstract Available.
  http://www.ncbi.nlm.nih.gov/entrez/query.fcgi?cmd=Retrieve&db=pubmed&dopt=Abstract&list_uids=5216477

- **Recovery of vision after bilateral arteritic central retinal artery occlusion.**
  Author(s): Riley AF, Aburn NS.
  Source: Clinical & Experimental Ophthalmology. 2004 April; 32(2): 226-8.
  http://www.ncbi.nlm.nih.gov/entrez/query.fcgi?cmd=Retrieve&db=pubmed&dopt=Abstract&list_uids=15068446

- **The role of disease-modifying antirheumatic drugs in the treatment of giant cell arteritis.**
  Author(s): Nuenninghoff DM, Matteson EL.
  Source: Clin Exp Rheumatol. 2003 November-December; 21(6 Suppl 32): S29-34. Review.
  http://www.ncbi.nlm.nih.gov/entrez/query.fcgi?cmd=Retrieve&db=pubmed&dopt=Abstract&list_uids=14740425

- **The types of headache that affect the elderly.**
  Author(s): Poser CM.
  Source: Geriatrics. 1976 September; 31(9): 103-6.
  http://www.ncbi.nlm.nih.gov/entrez/query.fcgi?cmd=Retrieve&db=pubmed&dopt=Abstract&list_uids=955413

- **Upper extremity revascularization. Axillary-brachial bypass for temporal arteritis.**
  Author(s): Kellar SJ.
  Source: Aorn Journal. 1992 September; 56(3): 435-41. Review.
  http://www.ncbi.nlm.nih.gov/entrez/query.fcgi?cmd=Retrieve&db=pubmed&dopt=Abstract&list_uids=1345250

- **Visual recovery in two patients after intravenous methylprednisolone treatment of central retinal artery occlusion secondary to giant-cell arteritis.**
  Author(s): Matzkin DC, Slamovits TL, Sachs R, Burde RM.
  Source: Ophthalmology. 1992 January; 99(1): 68-71.
  http://www.ncbi.nlm.nih.gov/entrez/query.fcgi?cmd=Retrieve&db=pubmed&dopt=Abstract&list_uids=1741143

Additional Web Resources

A number of additional Web sites offer encyclopedic information covering CAM and related topics. The following is a representative sample:

- Alternative Medicine Foundation, Inc.: **http://www.herbmed.org/**

- AOL: **http://search.aol.com/cat.adp?id=169&layer=&from=subcats**

- Chinese Medicine: **http://www.newcenturynutrition.com/**

- drkoop.com®: **http://www.drkoop.com/InteractiveMedicine/IndexC.html**

- Family Village: **http://www.familyvillage.wisc.edu/med_altn.htm**

- Google: **http://directory.google.com/Top/Health/Alternative/**

- Healthnotes: **http://www.healthnotes.com/**

- MedWebPlus:
  http://medwebplus.com/subject/Alternative_and_Complementary_Medicine

- Open Directory Project: **http://dmoz.org/Health/Alternative/**

- HealthGate: **http://www.tnp.com/**

- WebMD®Health: **http://my.webmd.com/drugs_and_herbs**

- WholeHealthMD.com: **http://www.wholehealthmd.com/reflib/0,1529,00.html**

- Yahoo.com: **http://dir.yahoo.com/Health/Alternative_Medicine/**

General References

A good place to find general background information on CAM is the National Library of Medicine. It has prepared within the MEDLINEplus system an information topic page dedicated to complementary and alternative medicine. To access this page, go to the MEDLINEplus site at **http://www.nlm.nih.gov/medlineplus/alternativemedicine.html**. This Web site provides a general overview of various topics and can lead to a number of general sources.

CHAPTER 4. BOOKS ON GIANT CELL ARTERITIS

Overview

This chapter provides bibliographic book references relating to giant cell arteritis. In addition to online booksellers such as **www.amazon.com** and **www.bn.com**, excellent sources for book titles on giant cell arteritis include the Combined Health Information Database and the National Library of Medicine. Your local medical library also may have these titles available for loan.

Book Summaries: Federal Agencies

The Combined Health Information Database collects various book abstracts from a variety of healthcare institutions and federal agencies. To access these summaries, go directly to the following hyperlink: **http://chid.nih.gov/detail/detail.html**. You will need to use the "Detailed Search" option. To find book summaries, use the drop boxes at the bottom of the search page where "You may refine your search by." Select the dates and language you prefer. For the format option, select "Monograph/Book." Now type "giant cell arteritis" (or synonyms) into the "For these words:" box. You should check back periodically with this database which is updated every three months. The following is a typical result when searching for books on giant cell arteritis:

- **Diseases of the Oral Mucosa and the Lips**

  Source: Orlando, FL: W.B. Saunders Company. 1993. 389 p.

  Contact: Available from W.B. Saunders Company. Order Fulfillment, 6277 Sea Harbor Drive, Orlando, FL 32887-4430. (800) 545-2522 (individuals) or (800) 782-4479 (schools); Fax (800) 874-6418 or (407) 352-3445; http://www.wbsaunders.com. PRICE: $99.00 plus shipping and handling. ISBN: 0721640397.

  Summary: This book is a clinically oriented atlas and text covering the symptoms and diseases of the oral mucosa and perioral skin. The authors focus on the essential aspects of each illness, concentrating on the clinical features that are important in the differential diagnosis. The authors include not only diseases confined to the oral mucosa but also those oral problems that may be signs of accompanying cutaneous (skin) or systemic diseases. Sixty-seven chapters are presented in three sections: the normal oral mucosa, general aspects of oral pathology, and diseases of the oral mucosa and the lips. Specific topics are inflammation of the lips, acquired diseases of the tongue, gingival hyperplasia, enlargement of the parotid gland, aphthous ulcers (stomatitis), pyostomatitis vegetans, disorders of pigmentation, urticaria and angioedema, psoriasis, Reiter's syndrome, lichen planus, graft-versus-host disease, rosacea, perioral dermatitis, erythema multiforme, acute febrile neutrophilic dermatosis (Sweet's syndrome), vesicular and bullous autoimmune diseases, desquamative gingivitis, necrotizing sialometaplasia, oral mucosal hemorrhage, viral diseases, bacterial diseases, fungal diseases, protozoal and parasitic diseases, mechanical damage, trauma, allergic and toxic contact stomatitis, occupational diseases of the oral mucosa, drug reactions and side effects, morphea and scleroderma, lichen sclerosus et atrophicus, dermatomyositis, lupus erythematosus, Sjogren's syndrome, polyarteritis nodosa, **giant cell arteritis,** plasma cell gingivitis, oral submucous fibrosis, halitosis, xerostomia, sialorrhea, self-induced mucosal injuries, benign granulomatous processes, malignant granulomatoses, heterotopias and congenital malformations, genodermatoses and congenital syndromes, benign and malignant tumors, actinic keratosis, leukoplakia, paraneoplastic disorders, and oral signs of hematologic, nutritional, metabolic, and endocrine disorders. Each chapter includes full-color photographs and references are provided in individual sections. A subject index concludes the volume. (AA-M).

Chapters on Giant Cell Arteritis

In order to find chapters that specifically relate to giant cell arteritis, an excellent source of abstracts is the Combined Health Information Database. You will need to limit your search to book chapters and giant cell arteritis using the "Detailed Search" option. Go to the following hyperlink: **http://chid.nih.gov/detail/detail.html.** To find book chapters, use the drop boxes at the bottom of the search page where "You may refine your search by." Select the dates and language you prefer, and the format option "Book Chapter." Type "giant cell arteritis" (or synonyms) into the "For these words:" box. The following is a typical result when searching for book chapters on giant cell arteritis:

- **Giant Cell Arteritis (Temporal Arteritis)**

  Source: in Bork, K., et al. Diseases of the Oral Mucosa and the Lips. Philadelphia, PA: W.B. Saunders Company. 1993. p. 218-219.

  Contact: Available from W.B. Saunders Company. Book Orders Fulfillment Department, 6277 Sea Harbor Drive, Orlando, FL 32821-9854. (800) 545-2522. Fax (800) 874-6418 or (407) 352-3445. Website: www.wbsaunders.com. PRICE: $95.00 plus shipping and handling. ISBN: 0721640397.

  Summary: This chapter on **giant cell arteritis,** or **temporal arteritis,** is from a textbook of diseases of the oral mucosa and the lips. **Giant cell arteritis** is a widespread inflammatory arteritis. The disease is found mainly in older women and is closely related to polymyalgia rheumatica. The chapter covers the clinical features, oral features, diagnosis, and therapy of **giant cell arteritis.** The most common clinical feature is a sharp unilateral headache concentrated on the temple. Another common finding is claudication of the jaw muscle on chewing. The crucial problem is involvement of the central artery of the optic nerve leading to initially transitory but eventually permanent blindness. The most common oral finding is unilateral tongue necrosis. Initially the patient has episodes of unilateral tongue pain and difficulty speaking. There may also be episodes of pallor due to the insufficient blood supply to the tongue. As the process progresses (and this may occur very rapidly), the artery closes, leading to infarction and necrosis (tissue death). The necrosis of the tongue produces a large, heavily coated ulcer that heals slowly over months. Despite the amazing regenerative ability of the oral cavity, scarring and impaired function are to be expected. Treatment involves high doses of oral or intravenous corticosteroids. Once improvement is obtained, a lower maintenance dose, often even alternate day therapy, can control the disorder. 1 figure. 16 references.

APPENDICES

APPENDIX A. PHYSICIAN RESOURCES

Overview

In this chapter, we focus on databases and Internet-based guidelines and information resources created or written for a professional audience.

NIH Guidelines

Commonly referred to as "clinical" or "professional" guidelines, the National Institutes of Health publish physician guidelines for the most common diseases. Publications are available at the following by relevant Institute[8]:

- Office of the Director (OD); guidelines consolidated across agencies available at http://www.nih.gov/health/consumer/conkey.htm

- National Institute of General Medical Sciences (NIGMS); fact sheets available at http://www.nigms.nih.gov/news/facts/

- National Library of Medicine (NLM); extensive encyclopedia (A.D.A.M., Inc.) with guidelines: http://www.nlm.nih.gov/medlineplus/healthtopics.html

- National Cancer Institute (NCI); guidelines available at http://www.cancer.gov/cancerinfo/list.aspx?viewid=5f35036e-5497-4d86-8c2c-714a9f7c8d25

- National Eye Institute (NEI); guidelines available at http://www.nei.nih.gov/order/index.htm

- National Heart, Lung, and Blood Institute (NHLBI); guidelines available at http://www.nhlbi.nih.gov/guidelines/index.htm

- National Human Genome Research Institute (NHGRI); research available at http://www.genome.gov/page.cfm?pageID=10000375

- National Institute on Aging (NIA); guidelines available at http://www.nia.nih.gov/health/

---

[8] These publications are typically written by one or more of the various NIH Institutes.

- National Institute on Alcohol Abuse and Alcoholism (NIAAA); guidelines available at http://www.niaaa.nih.gov/publications/publications.htm

- National Institute of Allergy and Infectious Diseases (NIAID); guidelines available at http://www.niaid.nih.gov/publications/

- National Institute of Arthritis and Musculoskeletal and Skin Diseases (NIAMS); fact sheets and guidelines available at http://www.niams.nih.gov/hi/index.htm

- National Institute of Child Health and Human Development (NICHD); guidelines available at http://www.nichd.nih.gov/publications/pubskey.cfm

- National Institute on Deafness and Other Communication Disorders (NIDCD); fact sheets and guidelines at http://www.nidcd.nih.gov/health/

- National Institute of Dental and Craniofacial Research (NIDCR); guidelines available at http://www.nidr.nih.gov/health/

- National Institute of Diabetes and Digestive and Kidney Diseases (NIDDK); guidelines available at http://www.niddk.nih.gov/health/health.htm

- National Institute on Drug Abuse (NIDA); guidelines available at http://www.nida.nih.gov/DrugAbuse.html

- National Institute of Environmental Health Sciences (NIEHS); environmental health information available at http://www.niehs.nih.gov/external/facts.htm

- National Institute of Mental Health (NIMH); guidelines available at http://www.nimh.nih.gov/practitioners/index.cfm

- National Institute of Neurological Disorders and Stroke (NINDS); neurological disorder information pages available at http://www.ninds.nih.gov/health_and_medical/disorder_index.htm

- National Institute of Nursing Research (NINR); publications on selected illnesses at http://www.nih.gov/ninr/news-info/publications.html

- National Institute of Biomedical Imaging and Bioengineering; general information at http://grants.nih.gov/grants/becon/becon_info.htm

- Center for Information Technology (CIT); referrals to other agencies based on keyword searches available at http://kb.nih.gov/www_query_main.asp

- National Center for Complementary and Alternative Medicine (NCCAM); health information available at http://nccam.nih.gov/health/

- National Center for Research Resources (NCRR); various information directories available at http://www.ncrr.nih.gov/publications.asp

- Office of Rare Diseases; various fact sheets available at http://rarediseases.info.nih.gov/html/resources/rep_pubs.html

- Centers for Disease Control and Prevention; various fact sheets on infectious diseases available at http://www.cdc.gov/publications.htm

NIH Databases

In addition to the various Institutes of Health that publish professional guidelines, the NIH has designed a number of databases for professionals.[9] Physician-oriented resources provide a wide variety of information related to the biomedical and health sciences, both past and present. The format of these resources varies. Searchable databases, bibliographic citations, full-text articles (when available), archival collections, and images are all available. The following are referenced by the National Library of Medicine:[10]

- **Bioethics:** Access to published literature on the ethical, legal, and public policy issues surrounding healthcare and biomedical research. This information is provided in conjunction with the Kennedy Institute of Ethics located at Georgetown University, Washington, D.C.: **http://www.nlm.nih.gov/databases/databases_bioethics.html**

- **HIV/AIDS Resources:** Describes various links and databases dedicated to HIV/AIDS research: **http://www.nlm.nih.gov/pubs/factsheets/aidsinfs.html**

- **NLM Online Exhibitions:** Describes "Exhibitions in the History of Medicine": **http://www.nlm.nih.gov/exhibition/exhibition.html**. Additional resources for historical scholarship in medicine: **http://www.nlm.nih.gov/hmd/hmd.html**

- **Biotechnology Information:** Access to public databases. The National Center for Biotechnology Information conducts research in computational biology, develops software tools for analyzing genome data, and disseminates biomedical information for the better understanding of molecular processes affecting human health and disease: **http://www.ncbi.nlm.nih.gov/**

- **Population Information:** The National Library of Medicine provides access to worldwide coverage of population, family planning, and related health issues, including family planning technology and programs, fertility, and population law and policy: **http://www.nlm.nih.gov/databases/databases_population.html**

- **Cancer Information:** Access to cancer-oriented databases: **http://www.nlm.nih.gov/databases/databases_cancer.html**

- **Profiles in Science:** Offering the archival collections of prominent twentieth-century biomedical scientists to the public through modern digital technology: **http://www.profiles.nlm.nih.gov/**

- **Chemical Information:** Provides links to various chemical databases and references: **http://sis.nlm.nih.gov/Chem/ChemMain.html**

- **Clinical Alerts:** Reports the release of findings from the NIH-funded clinical trials where such release could significantly affect morbidity and mortality: **http://www.nlm.nih.gov/databases/alerts/clinical_alerts.html**

- **Space Life Sciences:** Provides links and information to space-based research (including NASA): **http://www.nlm.nih.gov/databases/databases_space.html**

- **MEDLINE:** Bibliographic database covering the fields of medicine, nursing, dentistry, veterinary medicine, the healthcare system, and the pre-clinical sciences: **http://www.nlm.nih.gov/databases/databases_medline.html**

---

[9] Remember, for the general public, the National Library of Medicine recommends the databases referenced in MEDLINE*plus* (**http://medlineplus.gov/** or **http://www.nlm.nih.gov/medlineplus/databases.html**).

[10] See **http://www.nlm.nih.gov/databases/databases.html**.

- **Toxicology and Environmental Health Information (TOXNET):** Databases covering toxicology and environmental health: **http://sis.nlm.nih.gov/Tox/ToxMain.html**

- **Visible Human Interface:** Anatomically detailed, three-dimensional representations of normal male and female human bodies: **http://www.nlm.nih.gov/research/visible/visible_human.html**

The NLM Gateway[11]

The NLM (National Library of Medicine) Gateway is a Web-based system that lets users search simultaneously in multiple retrieval systems at the U.S. National Library of Medicine (NLM). It allows users of NLM services to initiate searches from one Web interface, providing one-stop searching for many of NLM's information resources or databases.[12] To use the NLM Gateway, simply go to the search site at **http://gateway.nlm.nih.gov/gw/Cmd**. Type "giant cell arteritis" (or synonyms) into the search box and click "Search." The results will be presented in a tabular form, indicating the number of references in each database category.

Results Summary

Category	Items Found
Journal Articles	3823
Books / Periodicals / Audio Visual	12
Consumer Health	29
Meeting Abstracts	0
Other Collections	4
Total	3868

HSTAT[13]

HSTAT is a free, Web-based resource that provides access to full-text documents used in healthcare decision-making.[14] These documents include clinical practice guidelines, quick-reference guides for clinicians, consumer health brochures, evidence reports and technology assessments from the Agency for Healthcare Research and Quality (AHRQ), as well as AHRQ's Put Prevention Into Practice.[15] Simply search by "giant cell arteritis" (or synonyms) at the following Web site: **http://text.nlm.nih.gov**.

---

[11] Adapted from NLM: **http://gateway.nlm.nih.gov/gw/Cmd?Overview.x**.

[12] The NLM Gateway is currently being developed by the Lister Hill National Center for Biomedical Communications (LHNCBC) at the National Library of Medicine (NLM) of the National Institutes of Health (NIH).

[13] Adapted from HSTAT: **http://www.nlm.nih.gov/pubs/factsheets/hstat.html**.

[14] The HSTAT URL is **http://hstat.nlm.nih.gov/**.

[15] Other important documents in HSTAT include: the National Institutes of Health (NIH) Consensus Conference Reports and Technology Assessment Reports; the HIV/AIDS Treatment Information Service (ATIS) resource documents; the Substance Abuse and Mental Health Services Administration's Center for Substance Abuse Treatment (SAMHSA/CSAT) Treatment Improvement Protocols (TIP) and Center for Substance Abuse Prevention (SAMHSA/CSAP) Prevention Enhancement Protocols System (PEPS); the Public Health Service (PHS) Preventive Services Task Force's *Guide to Clinical Preventive Services*; the independent, nonfederal Task Force on Community Services' *Guide to Community Preventive Services*; and the Health Technology Advisory Committee (HTAC) of the Minnesota Health Care Commission (MHCC) health technology evaluations.

Coffee Break: Tutorials for Biologists[16]

Coffee Break is a general healthcare site that takes a scientific view of the news and covers recent breakthroughs in biology that may one day assist physicians in developing treatments. Here you will find a collection of short reports on recent biological discoveries. Each report incorporates interactive tutorials that demonstrate how bioinformatics tools are used as a part of the research process. Currently, all Coffee Breaks are written by NCBI staff.[17] Each report is about 400 words and is usually based on a discovery reported in one or more articles from recently published, peer-reviewed literature.[18] This site has new articles every few weeks, so it can be considered an online magazine of sorts. It is intended for general background information. You can access the Coffee Break Web site at the following hyperlink: **http://www.ncbi.nlm.nih.gov/Coffeebreak/**.

Other Commercial Databases

In addition to resources maintained by official agencies, other databases exist that are commercial ventures addressing medical professionals. Here are some examples that may interest you:

- **CliniWeb International:** Index and table of contents to selected clinical information on the Internet; see **http://www.ohsu.edu/cliniweb/**.

- **Medical World Search:** Searches full text from thousands of selected medical sites on the Internet; see **http://www.mwsearch.com/**.

---

[16] Adapted from **http://www.ncbi.nlm.nih.gov/Coffeebreak/Archive/FAQ.html**.

[17] The figure that accompanies each article is frequently supplied by an expert external to NCBI, in which case the source of the figure is cited. The result is an interactive tutorial that tells a biological story.

[18] After a brief introduction that sets the work described into a broader context, the report focuses on how a molecular understanding can provide explanations of observed biology and lead to therapies for diseases. Each vignette is accompanied by a figure and hypertext links that lead to a series of pages that interactively show how NCBI tools and resources are used in the research process.

APPENDIX B. PATIENT RESOURCES

Overview

Official agencies, as well as federally funded institutions supported by national grants, frequently publish a variety of guidelines written with the patient in mind. These are typically called "Fact Sheets" or "Guidelines." They can take the form of a brochure, information kit, pamphlet, or flyer. Often they are only a few pages in length. Since new guidelines on giant cell arteritis can appear at any moment and be published by a number of sources, the best approach to finding guidelines is to systematically scan the Internet-based services that post them.

Patient Guideline Sources

The remainder of this chapter directs you to sources which either publish or can help you find additional guidelines on topics related to giant cell arteritis. Due to space limitations, these sources are listed in a concise manner. Do not hesitate to consult the following sources by either using the Internet hyperlink provided, or, in cases where the contact information is provided, contacting the publisher or author directly.

The National Institutes of Health

The NIH gateway to patients is located at **http://health.nih.gov/**. From this site, you can search across various sources and institutes, a number of which are summarized below.

Topic Pages: MEDLINEplus

The National Library of Medicine has created a vast and patient-oriented healthcare information portal called MEDLINEplus. Within this Internet-based system are "health topic pages" which list links to available materials relevant to giant cell arteritis. To access this system, log on to **http://www.nlm.nih.gov/medlineplus/healthtopics.html**. From there you can either search using the alphabetical index or browse by broad topic areas. Recently, MEDLINEplus listed the following when searched for "giant cell arteritis":

Alzheimer's Disease
http://www.nlm.nih.gov/medlineplus/alzheimersdisease.html

Autoimmune Diseases
http://www.nlm.nih.gov/medlineplus/autoimmunediseases.html

Behcet's Syndrome
http://www.nlm.nih.gov/medlineplus/behcetssyndrome.html

Dementia
http://www.nlm.nih.gov/medlineplus/dementia.html

Eye Diseases
http://www.nlm.nih.gov/medlineplus/eyediseases.html

Heart Diseases
http://www.nlm.nih.gov/medlineplus/heartdiseases.html

Lupus
http://www.nlm.nih.gov/medlineplus/lupus.html

Myositis
http://www.nlm.nih.gov/medlineplus/myositis.html

Neurologic Diseases
http://www.nlm.nih.gov/medlineplus/neurologicdiseases.html

Paget's Disease of Bone
http://www.nlm.nih.gov/medlineplus/pagetsdiseaseofbone.html

Parkinson's Disease
http://www.nlm.nih.gov/medlineplus/parkinsonsdisease.html

Polymyalgia Rheumatica
http://www.nlm.nih.gov/medlineplus/polymyalgiarheumatica.html

Rheumatoid Arthritis
http://www.nlm.nih.gov/medlineplus/rheumatoidarthritis.html

Vasculitis
http://www.nlm.nih.gov/medlineplus/vasculitis.html

Within the health topic page dedicated to giant cell arteritis, the following was listed:

- Diagnosis/Symptoms

    ESR (Erythrocyte Sedimentation Rate): Sed Rate
    Source: American Association for Clinical Chemistry
    http://www.labtestsonline.org/understanding/analytes/esr/test.html

- Treatment

    Prednisone
    Source: Myasthenia Gravis Foundation of America
    http://www.myasthenia.org/information/prednisone.pdf

- From the National Institutes of Health

  Questions and Answers about Polymyalgia Rheumatica and Giant Cell Arteritis
  Source: National Institute of Arthritis and Musculoskeletal and Skin Diseases
  http://www.niams.nih.gov/hi/topics/polymyalgia/index.htm

- Organizations

  American College of Rheumatology
  http://www.rheumatology.org/

  Arthritis Foundation
  http://www.arthritis.org/

  National Institute of Arthritis and Musculoskeletal and Skin Diseases
  http://www.niams.nih.gov/

- Research

  Giant-Cell Arteritis and Polymyalgia Rheumatica
  Source: American College of Physicians
  http://www.annals.org/cgi/content/full/139/6/I-55

You may also choose to use the search utility provided by MEDLINEplus at the following Web address: **http://www.nlm.nih.gov/medlineplus/**. Simply type a keyword into the search box and click "Search." This utility is similar to the NIH search utility, with the exception that it only includes materials that are linked within the MEDLINEplus system (mostly patient-oriented information). It also has the disadvantage of generating unstructured results. We recommend, therefore, that you use this method only if you have a very targeted search.

The NIH Search Utility

The NIH search utility allows you to search for documents on over 100 selected Web sites that comprise the NIH-WEB-SPACE. Each of these servers is "crawled" and indexed on an ongoing basis. Your search will produce a list of various documents, all of which will relate in some way to giant cell arteritis. The drawbacks of this approach are that the information is not organized by theme and that the references are often a mix of information for professionals and patients. Nevertheless, a large number of the listed Web sites provide useful background information. We can only recommend this route, therefore, for relatively rare or specific disorders, or when using highly targeted searches. To use the NIH search utility, visit the following Web page: **http://search.nih.gov/index.html**.

Additional Web Sources

A number of Web sites are available to the public that often link to government sites. These can also point you in the direction of essential information. The following is a representative sample:

- AOL: **http://search.aol.com/cat.adp?id=168&layer=&from=subcats**

- Family Village: **http://www.familyvillage.wisc.edu/specific.htm**

- Google: **http://directory.google.com/Top/Health/Conditions_and_Diseases/**

- Med Help International: **http://www.medhelp.org/HealthTopics/A.html**

- Open Directory Project: **http://dmoz.org/Health/Conditions_and_Diseases/**

- Yahoo.com: **http://dir.yahoo.com/Health/Diseases_and_Conditions/**

- WebMD®Health: **http://my.webmd.com/health_topics**

Finding Associations

There are several Internet directories that provide lists of medical associations with information on or resources relating to giant cell arteritis. By consulting all of associations listed in this chapter, you will have nearly exhausted all sources for patient associations concerned with giant cell arteritis.

The National Health Information Center (NHIC)

The National Health Information Center (NHIC) offers a free referral service to help people find organizations that provide information about giant cell arteritis. For more information, see the NHIC's Web site at **http://www.health.gov/NHIC/** or contact an information specialist by calling 1-800-336-4797.

Directory of Health Organizations

The Directory of Health Organizations, provided by the National Library of Medicine Specialized Information Services, is a comprehensive source of information on associations. The Directory of Health Organizations database can be accessed via the Internet at **http://www.sis.nlm.nih.gov/Dir/DirMain.html**. It is composed of two parts: DIRLINE and Health Hotlines.

The DIRLINE database comprises some 10,000 records of organizations, research centers, and government institutes and associations that primarily focus on health and biomedicine. To access DIRLINE directly, go to the following Web site: **http://dirline.nlm.nih.gov/**. Simply type in "giant cell arteritis" (or a synonym), and you will receive information on all relevant organizations listed in the database.

Health Hotlines directs you to toll-free numbers to over 300 organizations. You can access this database directly at **http://www.sis.nlm.nih.gov/hotlines/**. On this page, you are given the option to search by keyword or by browsing the subject list. When you have received your search results, click on the name of the organization for its description and contact information.

The Combined Health Information Database

Another comprehensive source of information on healthcare associations is the Combined Health Information Database. Using the "Detailed Search" option, you will need to limit your search to "Organizations" and "giant cell arteritis". Type the following hyperlink into your Web browser: **http://chid.nih.gov/detail/detail.html**. To find associations, use the drop boxes at the bottom of the search page where "You may refine your search by." For publication date, select "All Years." Then, select your preferred language and the format option "Organization Resource Sheet." Type "giant cell arteritis" (or synonyms) into the "For these words:" box. You should check back periodically with this database since it is updated every three months.

The National Organization for Rare Disorders, Inc.

The National Organization for Rare Disorders, Inc. has prepared a Web site that provides, at no charge, lists of associations organized by health topic. You can access this database at the following Web site: **http://www.rarediseases.org/search/orgsearch.html**. Type "giant cell arteritis" (or a synonym) into the search box, and click "Submit Query."

APPENDIX C. FINDING MEDICAL LIBRARIES

Overview

In this Appendix, we show you how to quickly find a medical library in your area.

Preparation

Your local public library and medical libraries have interlibrary loan programs with the National Library of Medicine (NLM), one of the largest medical collections in the world. According to the NLM, most of the literature in the general and historical collections of the National Library of Medicine is available on interlibrary loan to any library. If you would like to access NLM medical literature, then visit a library in your area that can request the publications for you.[19]

Finding a Local Medical Library

The quickest method to locate medical libraries is to use the Internet-based directory published by the National Network of Libraries of Medicine (NN/LM). This network includes 4626 members and affiliates that provide many services to librarians, health professionals, and the public. To find a library in your area, simply visit **http://nnlm.gov/members/adv.html** or call 1-800-338-7657.

Medical Libraries in the U.S. and Canada

In addition to the NN/LM, the National Library of Medicine (NLM) lists a number of libraries with reference facilities that are open to the public. The following is the NLM's list and includes hyperlinks to each library's Web site. These Web pages can provide information on hours of operation and other restrictions. The list below is a small sample of

---

[19] Adapted from the NLM: **http://www.nlm.nih.gov/psd/cas/interlibrary.html**.

libraries recommended by the National Library of Medicine (sorted alphabetically by name of the U.S. state or Canadian province where the library is located)[20]:

- **Alabama:** Health InfoNet of Jefferson County (Jefferson County Library Cooperative, Lister Hill Library of the Health Sciences), **http://www.uab.edu/infonet/**

- **Alabama:** Richard M. Scrushy Library (American Sports Medicine Institute)

- **Arizona:** Samaritan Regional Medical Center: The Learning Center (Samaritan Health System, Phoenix, Arizona), **http://www.samaritan.edu/library/bannerlibs.htm**

- **California:** Kris Kelly Health Information Center (St. Joseph Health System, Humboldt), **http://www.humboldt1.com/~kkhic/index.html**

- **California:** Community Health Library of Los Gatos, **http://www.healthlib.org/orgresources.html**

- **California:** Consumer Health Program and Services (CHIPS) (County of Los Angeles Public Library, Los Angeles County Harbor-UCLA Medical Center Library) - Carson, CA, **http://www.colapublib.org/services/chips.html**

- **California:** Gateway Health Library (Sutter Gould Medical Foundation)

- **California:** Health Library (Stanford University Medical Center), **http://www-med.stanford.edu/healthlibrary/**

- **California:** Patient Education Resource Center - Health Information and Resources (University of California, San Francisco), **http://sfghdean.ucsf.edu/barnett/PERC/default.asp**

- **California:** Redwood Health Library (Petaluma Health Care District), **http://www.phcd.org/rdwdlib.html**

- **California:** Los Gatos PlaneTree Health Library, **http://planetreesanjose.org/**

- **California:** Sutter Resource Library (Sutter Hospitals Foundation, Sacramento), **http://suttermedicalcenter.org/library/**

- **California:** Health Sciences Libraries (University of California, Davis), **http://www.lib.ucdavis.edu/healthsci/**

- **California:** ValleyCare Health Library & Ryan Comer Cancer Resource Center (ValleyCare Health System, Pleasanton), **http://gaelnet.stmarys-ca.edu/other.libs/gbal/east/vchl.html**

- **California:** Washington Community Health Resource Library (Fremont), **http://www.healthlibrary.org/**

- **Colorado:** William V. Gervasini Memorial Library (Exempla Healthcare), **http://www.saintjosephdenver.org/yourhealth/libraries/**

- **Connecticut:** Hartford Hospital Health Science Libraries (Hartford Hospital), **http://www.harthosp.org/library/**

- **Connecticut:** Healthnet: Connecticut Consumer Health Information Center (University of Connecticut Health Center, Lyman Maynard Stowe Library), **http://library.uchc.edu/departm/hnet/**

---

[20] Abstracted from **http://www.nlm.nih.gov/medlineplus/libraries.html**.

- **Connecticut:** Waterbury Hospital Health Center Library (Waterbury Hospital, Waterbury), http://www.waterburyhospital.com/library/consumer.shtml

- **Delaware:** Consumer Health Library (Christiana Care Health System, Eugene du Pont Preventive Medicine & Rehabilitation Institute, Wilmington), http://www.christianacare.org/health_guide/health_guide_pmri_health_info.cfm

- **Delaware:** Lewis B. Flinn Library (Delaware Academy of Medicine, Wilmington), http://www.delamed.org/chls.html

- **Georgia:** Family Resource Library (Medical College of Georgia, Augusta), http://cmc.mcg.edu/kids_families/fam_resources/fam_res_lib/frl.htm

- **Georgia:** Health Resource Center (Medical Center of Central Georgia, Macon), http://www.mccg.org/hrc/hrchome.asp

- **Hawaii:** Hawaii Medical Library: Consumer Health Information Service (Hawaii Medical Library, Honolulu), http://hml.org/CHIS/

- **Idaho:** DeArmond Consumer Health Library (Kootenai Medical Center, Coeur d'Alene), http://www.nicon.org/DeArmond/index.htm

- **Illinois:** Health Learning Center of Northwestern Memorial Hospital (Chicago), http://www.nmh.org/health_info/hlc.html

- **Illinois:** Medical Library (OSF Saint Francis Medical Center, Peoria), http://www.osfsaintfrancis.org/general/library/

- **Kentucky:** Medical Library - Services for Patients, Families, Students & the Public (Central Baptist Hospital, Lexington), http://www.centralbap.com/education/community/library.cfm

- **Kentucky:** University of Kentucky - Health Information Library (Chandler Medical Center, Lexington), http://www.mc.uky.edu/PatientEd/

- **Louisiana:** Alton Ochsner Medical Foundation Library (Alton Ochsner Medical Foundation, New Orleans), http://www.ochsner.org/library/

- **Louisiana:** Louisiana State University Health Sciences Center Medical Library-Shreveport, http://lib-sh.lsuhsc.edu/

- **Maine:** Franklin Memorial Hospital Medical Library (Franklin Memorial Hospital, Farmington), http://www.fchn.org/fmh/lib.htm

- **Maine:** Gerrish-True Health Sciences Library (Central Maine Medical Center, Lewiston), http://www.cmmc.org/library/library.html

- **Maine:** Hadley Parrot Health Science Library (Eastern Maine Healthcare, Bangor), http://www.emh.org/hll/hpl/guide.htm

- **Maine:** Maine Medical Center Library (Maine Medical Center, Portland), http://www.mmc.org/library/

- **Maine:** Parkview Hospital (Brunswick), http://www.parkviewhospital.org/

- **Maine:** Southern Maine Medical Center Health Sciences Library (Southern Maine Medical Center, Biddeford), http://www.smmc.org/services/service.php3?choice=10

- **Maine:** Stephens Memorial Hospital's Health Information Library (Western Maine Health, Norway), http://www.wmhcc.org/Library/

- **Manitoba, Canada:** Consumer & Patient Health Information Service (University of Manitoba Libraries), http://www.umanitoba.ca/libraries/units/health/reference/chis.html

- **Manitoba, Canada:** J.W. Crane Memorial Library (Deer Lodge Centre, Winnipeg), http://www.deerlodge.mb.ca/crane_library/about.asp

- **Maryland:** Health Information Center at the Wheaton Regional Library (Montgomery County, Dept. of Public Libraries, Wheaton Regional Library), http://www.mont.lib.md.us/healthinfo/hic.asp

- **Massachusetts:** Baystate Medical Center Library (Baystate Health System), http://www.baystatehealth.com/1024/

- **Massachusetts:** Boston University Medical Center Alumni Medical Library (Boston University Medical Center), http://med-libwww.bu.edu/library/lib.html

- **Massachusetts:** Lowell General Hospital Health Sciences Library (Lowell General Hospital, Lowell), http://www.lowellgeneral.org/library/HomePageLinks/WWW.htm

- **Massachusetts:** Paul E. Woodard Health Sciences Library (New England Baptist Hospital, Boston), http://www.nebh.org/health_lib.asp

- **Massachusetts:** St. Luke's Hospital Health Sciences Library (St. Luke's Hospital, Southcoast Health System, New Bedford), http://www.southcoast.org/library/

- **Massachusetts:** Treadwell Library Consumer Health Reference Center (Massachusetts General Hospital), http://www.mgh.harvard.edu/library/chrcindex.html

- **Massachusetts:** UMass HealthNet (University of Massachusetts Medical School, Worchester), http://healthnet.umassmed.edu/

- **Michigan:** Botsford General Hospital Library - Consumer Health (Botsford General Hospital, Library & Internet Services), http://www.botsfordlibrary.org/consumer.htm

- **Michigan:** Helen DeRoy Medical Library (Providence Hospital and Medical Centers), http://www.providence-hospital.org/library/

- **Michigan:** Marquette General Hospital - Consumer Health Library (Marquette General Hospital, Health Information Center), http://www.mgh.org/center.html

- **Michigan:** Patient Education Resouce Center - University of Michigan Cancer Center (University of Michigan Comprehensive Cancer Center, Ann Arbor), http://www.cancer.med.umich.edu/learn/leares.htm

- **Michigan:** Sladen Library & Center for Health Information Resources - Consumer Health Information (Detroit), http://www.henryford.com/body.cfm?id=39330

- **Montana:** Center for Health Information (St. Patrick Hospital and Health Sciences Center, Missoula)

- **National:** Consumer Health Library Directory (Medical Library Association, Consumer and Patient Health Information Section), http://caphis.mlanet.org/directory/index.html

- **National:** National Network of Libraries of Medicine (National Library of Medicine) - provides library services for health professionals in the United States who do not have access to a medical library, http://nnlm.gov/

- **National:** NN/LM List of Libraries Serving the Public (National Network of Libraries of Medicine), http://nnlm.gov/members/

- **Nevada:** Health Science Library, West Charleston Library (Las Vegas-Clark County Library District, Las Vegas), http://www.lvccld.org/special_collections/medical/index.htm

- **New Hampshire:** Dartmouth Biomedical Libraries (Dartmouth College Library, Hanover), http://www.dartmouth.edu/~biomed/resources.htmld/conshealth.htmld/

- **New Jersey:** Consumer Health Library (Rahway Hospital, Rahway), http://www.rahwayhospital.com/library.htm

- **New Jersey:** Dr. Walter Phillips Health Sciences Library (Englewood Hospital and Medical Center, Englewood), http://www.englewoodhospital.com/links/index.htm

- **New Jersey:** Meland Foundation (Englewood Hospital and Medical Center, Englewood), http://www.geocities.com/ResearchTriangle/9360/

- **New York:** Choices in Health Information (New York Public Library) - NLM Consumer Pilot Project participant, http://www.nypl.org/branch/health/links.html

- **New York:** Health Information Center (Upstate Medical University, State University of New York, Syracuse), http://www.upstate.edu/library/hic/

- **New York:** Health Sciences Library (Long Island Jewish Medical Center, New Hyde Park), http://www.lij.edu/library/library.html

- **New York:** ViaHealth Medical Library (Rochester General Hospital), http://www.nyam.org/library/

- **Ohio:** Consumer Health Library (Akron General Medical Center, Medical & Consumer Health Library), http://www.akrongeneral.org/hwlibrary.htm

- **Oklahoma:** The Health Information Center at Saint Francis Hospital (Saint Francis Health System, Tulsa), http://www.sfh-tulsa.com/services/healthinfo.asp

- **Oregon:** Planetree Health Resource Center (Mid-Columbia Medical Center, The Dalles), http://www.mcmc.net/phrc/

- **Pennsylvania:** Community Health Information Library (Milton S. Hershey Medical Center, Hershey), http://www.hmc.psu.edu/commhealth/

- **Pennsylvania:** Community Health Resource Library (Geisinger Medical Center, Danville), http://www.geisinger.edu/education/commlib.shtml

- **Pennsylvania:** HealthInfo Library (Moses Taylor Hospital, Scranton), http://www.mth.org/healthwellness.html

- **Pennsylvania:** Hopwood Library (University of Pittsburgh, Health Sciences Library System, Pittsburgh), http://www.hsls.pitt.edu/guides/chi/hopwood/index_html

- **Pennsylvania:** Koop Community Health Information Center (College of Physicians of Philadelphia), http://www.collphyphil.org/kooppg1.shtml

- **Pennsylvania:** Learning Resources Center - Medical Library (Susquehanna Health System, Williamsport), http://www.shscares.org/services/lrc/index.asp

- **Pennsylvania:** Medical Library (UPMC Health System, Pittsburgh), http://www.upmc.edu/passavant/library.htm

- **Quebec, Canada:** Medical Library (Montreal General Hospital), http://www.mghlib.mcgill.ca/

- **South Dakota:** Rapid City Regional Hospital Medical Library (Rapid City Regional Hospital), **http://www.rcrh.org/Services/Library/Default.asp**

- **Texas:** Houston HealthWays (Houston Academy of Medicine-Texas Medical Center Library), **http://hhw.library.tmc.edu/**

- **Washington:** Community Health Library (Kittitas Valley Community Hospital), **http://www.kvch.com/**

- **Washington:** Southwest Washington Medical Center Library (Southwest Washington Medical Center, Vancouver), **http://www.swmedicalcenter.com/body.cfm?id=72**

ONLINE GLOSSARIES

The Internet provides access to a number of free-to-use medical dictionaries. The National Library of Medicine has compiled the following list of online dictionaries:

- ADAM Medical Encyclopedia (A.D.A.M., Inc.), comprehensive medical reference: **http://www.nlm.nih.gov/medlineplus/encyclopedia.html**

- MedicineNet.com Medical Dictionary (MedicineNet, Inc.): **http://www.medterms.com/Script/Main/hp.asp**

- Merriam-Webster Medical Dictionary (Inteli-Health, Inc.): **http://www.intelihealth.com/IH/**

- Multilingual Glossary of Technical and Popular Medical Terms in Eight European Languages (European Commission) - Danish, Dutch, English, French, German, Italian, Portuguese, and Spanish: **http://allserv.rug.ac.be/~rvdstich/eugloss/welcome.html**

- On-line Medical Dictionary (CancerWEB): **http://cancerweb.ncl.ac.uk/omd/**

- Rare Diseases Terms (Office of Rare Diseases): **http://ord.aspensys.com/asp/diseases/diseases.asp**

- Technology Glossary (National Library of Medicine) - Health Care Technology: **http://www.nlm.nih.gov/nichsr/ta101/ta10108.htm**

Beyond these, MEDLINEplus contains a very patient-friendly encyclopedia covering every aspect of medicine (licensed from A.D.A.M., Inc.). The ADAM Medical Encyclopedia can be accessed at **http://www.nlm.nih.gov/medlineplus/encyclopedia.html**. ADAM is also available on commercial Web sites such as drkoop.com (**http://www.drkoop.com/**) and Web MD (**http://my.webmd.com/adam/asset/adam_disease_articles/a_to_z/a**).

Online Dictionary Directories

The following are additional online directories compiled by the National Library of Medicine, including a number of specialized medical dictionaries:

- Medical Dictionaries: Medical & Biological (World Health Organization): **http://www.who.int/hlt/virtuallibrary/English/diction.htm#Medical**

- MEL-Michigan Electronic Library List of Online Health and Medical Dictionaries (Michigan Electronic Library): **http://mel.lib.mi.us/health/health-dictionaries.html**

- Patient Education: Glossaries (DMOZ Open Directory Project): **http://dmoz.org/Health/Education/Patient_Education/Glossaries/**

- Web of Online Dictionaries (Bucknell University): **http://www.yourdictionary.com/diction5.html#medicine**

GIANT CELL ARTERITIS DICTIONARY

The definitions below are derived from official public sources, including the National Institutes of Health [NIH] and the European Union [EU].

Abscess: A localized, circumscribed collection of pus. [NIH]

Accommodation: Adjustment, especially that of the eye for various distances. [EU]

Acetylcholine: A neurotransmitter. Acetylcholine in vertebrates is the major transmitter at neuromuscular junctions, autonomic ganglia, parasympathetic effector junctions, a subset of sympathetic effector junctions, and at many sites in the central nervous system. It is generally not used as an administered drug because it is broken down very rapidly by cholinesterases, but it is useful in some ophthalmological applications. [NIH]

Actinic keratosis: A precancerous condition of thick, scaly patches of skin. Also called solar or senile keratosis. [NIH]

Adjuvant: A substance which aids another, such as an auxiliary remedy; in immunology, nonspecific stimulator (e.g., BCG vaccine) of the immune response. [EU]

Adrenal Cortex: The outer layer of the adrenal gland. It secretes mineralocorticoids, androgens, and glucocorticoids. [NIH]

Adrenal Glands: Paired glands situated in the retroperitoneal tissues at the superior pole of each kidney. [NIH]

Adverse Effect: An unwanted side effect of treatment. [NIH]

Algorithms: A procedure consisting of a sequence of algebraic formulas and/or logical steps to calculate or determine a given task. [NIH]

Alkalosis: A pathological condition that removes acid or adds base to the body fluids. [NIH]

Alleles: Mutually exclusive forms of the same gene, occupying the same locus on homologous chromosomes, and governing the same biochemical and developmental process. [NIH]

Alternative medicine: Practices not generally recognized by the medical community as standard or conventional medical approaches and used instead of standard treatments. Alternative medicine includes the taking of dietary supplements, megadose vitamins, and herbal preparations; the drinking of special teas; and practices such as massage therapy, magnet therapy, spiritual healing, and meditation. [NIH]

Amino acid: Any organic compound containing an amino (-NH2 and a carboxyl (- COOH) group. The 20 a-amino acids listed in the accompanying table are the amino acids from which proteins are synthesized by formation of peptide bonds during ribosomal translation of messenger RNA; all except glycine, which is not optically active, have the L configuration. Other amino acids occurring in proteins, such as hydroxyproline in collagen, are formed by posttranslational enzymatic modification of amino acids residues in polypeptide chains. There are also several important amino acids, such as the neurotransmitter y-aminobutyric acid, that have no relation to proteins. Abbreviated AA. [EU]

Amino Acid Sequence: The order of amino acids as they occur in a polypeptide chain. This is referred to as the primary structure of proteins. It is of fundamental importance in determining protein conformation. [NIH]

Amputation: Surgery to remove part or all of a limb or appendage. [NIH]

Amyloidosis: A group of diseases in which protein is deposited in specific organs (localized amyloidosis) or throughout the body (systemic amyloidosis). Amyloidosis may be either primary (with no known cause) or secondary (caused by another disease, including some types of cancer). Generally, primary amyloidosis affects the nerves, skin, tongue, joints, heart, and liver; secondary amyloidosis often affects the spleen, kidneys, liver, and adrenal glands. [NIH]

Analytes: A component of a test sample the presence of which has to be demonstrated. The term "analyte" includes where appropriate formed from the analyte during the analyses. [NIH]

Androgens: A class of sex hormones associated with the development and maintenance of the secondary male sex characteristics, sperm induction, and sexual differentiation. In addition to increasing virility and libido, they also increase nitrogen and water retention and stimulate skeletal growth. [NIH]

Aneurysm: A sac formed by the dilatation of the wall of an artery, a vein, or the heart. [NIH]

Angioedema: A vascular reaction involving the deep dermis or subcutaneous or submucal tissues, representing localized edema caused by dilatation and increased permeability of the capillaries, and characterized by development of giant wheals. [EU]

Angiogenesis: Blood vessel formation. Tumor angiogenesis is the growth of blood vessels from surrounding tissue to a solid tumor. This is caused by the release of chemicals by the tumor. [NIH]

Angiography: Radiography of blood vessels after injection of a contrast medium. [NIH]

Animal model: An animal with a disease either the same as or like a disease in humans. Animal models are used to study the development and progression of diseases and to test new treatments before they are given to humans. Animals with transplanted human cancers or other tissues are called xenograft models. [NIH]

Annealing: The spontaneous alignment of two single DNA strands to form a double helix. [NIH]

Antiallergic: Counteracting allergy or allergic conditions. [EU]

Antibacterial: A substance that destroys bacteria or suppresses their growth or reproduction. [EU]

Antibiotic: A drug used to treat infections caused by bacteria and other microorganisms. [NIH]

Antibodies: Immunoglobulin molecules having a specific amino acid sequence by virtue of which they interact only with the antigen that induced their synthesis in cells of the lymphoid series (especially plasma cells), or with an antigen closely related to it. [NIH]

Antibody: A type of protein made by certain white blood cells in response to a foreign substance (antigen). Each antibody can bind to only a specific antigen. The purpose of this binding is to help destroy the antigen. Antibodies can work in several ways, depending on the nature of the antigen. Some antibodies destroy antigens directly. Others make it easier for white blood cells to destroy the antigen. [NIH]

Antigen: Any substance which is capable, under appropriate conditions, of inducing a specific immune response and of reacting with the products of that response, that is, with specific antibody or specifically sensitized T-lymphocytes, or both. Antigens may be soluble substances, such as toxins and foreign proteins, or particulate, such as bacteria and tissue cells; however, only the portion of the protein or polysaccharide molecule known as the antigenic determinant (q.v.) combines with antibody or a specific receptor on a lymphocyte. Abbreviated Ag. [EU]

Antigen-presenting cell: APC. A cell that shows antigen on its surface to other cells of the immune system. This is an important part of an immune response. [NIH]

Anti-inflammatory: Having to do with reducing inflammation. [NIH]

Anti-Inflammatory Agents: Substances that reduce or suppress inflammation. [NIH]

Antimetabolite: A chemical that is very similar to one required in a normal biochemical reaction in cells. Antimetabolites can stop or slow down the reaction. [NIH]

Antineoplastic: Inhibiting or preventing the development of neoplasms, checking the maturation and proliferation of malignant cells. [EU]

Aorta: The main trunk of the systemic arteries. [NIH]

Aortic Aneurysm: Aneurysm of the aorta. [NIH]

Arginine: An essential amino acid that is physiologically active in the L-form. [NIH]

Arterial: Pertaining to an artery or to the arteries. [EU]

Arteries: The vessels carrying blood away from the heart. [NIH]

Arterioles: The smallest divisions of the arteries located between the muscular arteries and the capillaries. [NIH]

Arteritis: Inflammation of an artery. [NIH]

Artery: Vessel-carrying blood from the heart to various parts of the body. [NIH]

Ascites: Accumulation or retention of free fluid within the peritoneal cavity. [NIH]

Aspirin: A drug that reduces pain, fever, inflammation, and blood clotting. Aspirin belongs to the family of drugs called nonsteroidal anti-inflammatory agents. It is also being studied in cancer prevention. [NIH]

Atypical: Irregular; not conformable to the type; in microbiology, applied specifically to strains of unusual type. [EU]

Autoantibodies: Antibodies that react with self-antigens (autoantigens) of the organism that produced them. [NIH]

Autoantigens: Endogenous tissue constituents that have the ability to interact with autoantibodies and cause an immune response. [NIH]

Autoimmune disease: A condition in which the body recognizes its own tissues as foreign and directs an immune response against them. [NIH]

Axillary: Pertaining to the armpit area, including the lymph nodes that are located there. [NIH]

Axons: Nerve fibers that are capable of rapidly conducting impulses away from the neuron cell body. [NIH]

Bacteria: Unicellular prokaryotic microorganisms which generally possess rigid cell walls, multiply by cell division, and exhibit three principal forms: round or coccal, rodlike or bacillary, and spiral or spirochetal. [NIH]

Benign: Not cancerous; does not invade nearby tissue or spread to other parts of the body. [NIH]

Bilateral: Affecting both the right and left side of body. [NIH]

Bile: An emulsifying agent produced in the liver and secreted into the duodenum. Its composition includes bile acids and salts, cholesterol, and electrolytes. It aids digestion of fats in the duodenum. [NIH]

Biochemical: Relating to biochemistry; characterized by, produced by, or involving chemical reactions in living organisms. [EU]

Biopolymers: Polymers, such as proteins, DNA, RNA, or polysaccharides formed by any living organism. [NIH]

Bioprosthesis: Prosthesis, usually heart valve, composed of biological material and whose durability depends upon the stability of the material after pretreatment, rather than regeneration by host cell ingrowth. Durability is achieved 1) mechanically by the interposition of a cloth, usually polytetrafluoroethylene, between the host and the graft, and 2) chemically by stabilization of the tissue by intermolecular linking, usually with glutaraldehyde, after removal of antigenic components, or the use of reconstituted and restructured biopolymers. [NIH]

Biopsy: Removal and pathologic examination of specimens in the form of small pieces of tissue from the living body. [NIH]

Biotechnology: Body of knowledge related to the use of organisms, cells or cell-derived constituents for the purpose of developing products which are technically, scientifically and clinically useful. Alteration of biologic function at the molecular level (i.e., genetic engineering) is a central focus; laboratory methods used include transfection and cloning technologies, sequence and structure analysis algorithms, computer databases, and gene and protein structure function analysis and prediction. [NIH]

Blood pressure: The pressure of blood against the walls of a blood vessel or heart chamber. Unless there is reference to another location, such as the pulmonary artery or one of the heart chambers, it refers to the pressure in the systemic arteries, as measured, for example, in the forearm. [NIH]

Blood vessel: A tube in the body through which blood circulates. Blood vessels include a network of arteries, arterioles, capillaries, venules, and veins. [NIH]

Blot: To transfer DNA, RNA, or proteins to an immobilizing matrix such as nitrocellulose. [NIH]

Body Fluids: Liquid components of living organisms. [NIH]

Bone Marrow: The soft tissue filling the cavities of bones. Bone marrow exists in two types, yellow and red. Yellow marrow is found in the large cavities of large bones and consists mostly of fat cells and a few primitive blood cells. Red marrow is a hematopoietic tissue and is the site of production of erythrocytes and granular leukocytes. Bone marrow is made up of a framework of connective tissue containing branching fibers with the frame being filled with marrow cells. [NIH]

Bowel: The long tube-shaped organ in the abdomen that completes the process of digestion. There is both a small and a large bowel. Also called the intestine. [NIH]

Brachial: All the nerves from the arm are ripped from the spinal cord. [NIH]

Bradykinin: A nonapeptide messenger that is enzymatically produced from kallidin in the blood where it is a potent but short-lived agent of arteriolar dilation and increased capillary permeability. Bradykinin is also released from mast cells during asthma attacks, from gut walls as a gastrointestinal vasodilator, from damaged tissues as a pain signal, and may be a neurotransmitter. [NIH]

Buccal: Pertaining to or directed toward the cheek. In dental anatomy, used to refer to the buccal surface of a tooth. [EU]

Bullous: Pertaining to or characterized by bullae. [EU]

Bypass: A surgical procedure in which the doctor creates a new pathway for the flow of body fluids. [NIH]

Calcium: A basic element found in nearly all organized tissues. It is a member of the alkaline earth family of metals with the atomic symbol Ca, atomic number 20, and atomic weight 40. Calcium is the most abundant mineral in the body and combines with phosphorus to form calcium phosphate in the bones and teeth. It is essential for the normal functioning of nerves and muscles and plays a role in blood coagulation (as factor IV) and in many enzymatic processes. [NIH]

Capillary: Any one of the minute vessels that connect the arterioles and venules, forming a network in nearly all parts of the body. Their walls act as semipermeable membranes for the interchange of various substances, including fluids, between the blood and tissue fluid; called also vas capillare. [EU]

Carbohydrate: An aldehyde or ketone derivative of a polyhydric alcohol, particularly of the pentahydric and hexahydric alcohols. They are so named because the hydrogen and oxygen are usually in the proportion to form water, (CH2O)n. The most important carbohydrates are the starches, sugars, celluloses, and gums. They are classified into mono-, di-, tri-, poly- and heterosaccharides. [EU]

Carcinogenic: Producing carcinoma. [EU]

Carcinoma: Cancer that begins in the skin or in tissues that line or cover internal organs. [NIH]

Cardiac: Having to do with the heart. [NIH]

Cardiovascular: Having to do with the heart and blood vessels. [NIH]

Cardiovascular disease: Any abnormal condition characterized by dysfunction of the heart and blood vessels. CVD includes atherosclerosis (especially coronary heart disease, which can lead to heart attacks), cerebrovascular disease (e.g., stroke), and hypertension (high blood pressure). [NIH]

Carotene: The general name for a group of pigments found in green, yellow, and leafy vegetables, and yellow fruits. The pigments are fat-soluble, unsaturated aliphatic hydrocarbons functioning as provitamins and are converted to vitamin A through enzymatic processes in the intestinal wall. [NIH]

Carpal Tunnel Syndrome: A median nerve injury inside the carpal tunnel that results in symptoms of pain, numbness, tingling, clumsiness, and a lack of sweating, which can be caused by work with certain hand and wrist postures. [NIH]

Case report: A detailed report of the diagnosis, treatment, and follow-up of an individual patient. Case reports also contain some demographic information about the patient (for example, age, gender, ethnic origin). [NIH]

Case series: A group or series of case reports involving patients who were given similar treatment. Reports of case series usually contain detailed information about the individual patients. This includes demographic information (for example, age, gender, ethnic origin) and information on diagnosis, treatment, response to treatment, and follow-up after treatment. [NIH]

Caudal: Denoting a position more toward the cauda, or tail, than some specified point of reference; same as inferior, in human anatomy. [EU]

Causal: Pertaining to a cause; directed against a cause. [EU]

Cell: The individual unit that makes up all of the tissues of the body. All living things are made up of one or more cells. [NIH]

Cell Death: The termination of the cell's ability to carry out vital functions such as metabolism, growth, reproduction, responsiveness, and adaptability. [NIH]

Central Nervous System: The main information-processing organs of the nervous system, consisting of the brain, spinal cord, and meninges. [NIH]

Central Nervous System Infections: Pathogenic infections of the brain, spinal cord, and meninges. DNA virus infections; RNA virus infections; bacterial infections; mycoplasma infections; Spirochaetales infections; fungal infections; protozoan infections; helminthiasis; and prion diseases may involve the central nervous system as a primary or secondary process. [NIH]

Central retinal artery: The blood vessel that carries blood into eye; supplies nutrition to the retina. [NIH]

Cerebellum: Part of the metencephalon that lies in the posterior cranial fossa behind the brain stem. It is concerned with the coordination of movement. [NIH]

Cerebral: Of or pertaining of the cerebrum or the brain. [EU]

Cerebral Arteries: The arteries supplying the cerebral cortex. [NIH]

Cerebrovascular: Pertaining to the blood vessels of the cerebrum, or brain. [EU]

Cerebrum: The largest part of the brain. It is divided into two hemispheres, or halves, called the cerebral hemispheres. The cerebrum controls muscle functions of the body and also controls speech, emotions, reading, writing, and learning. [NIH]

Chimera: An individual that contains cell populations derived from different zygotes. [NIH]

Cholesterol: The principal sterol of all higher animals, distributed in body tissues, especially the brain and spinal cord, and in animal fats and oils. [NIH]

Chromatin: The material of chromosomes. It is a complex of DNA, histones, and nonhistone proteins (chromosomal proteins, non-histone) found within the nucleus of a cell. [NIH]

Chronic: A disease or condition that persists or progresses over a long period of time. [NIH]

Chronic Disease: Disease or ailment of long duration. [NIH]

Chronic lymphocytic leukemia: A slowly progressing disease in which too many white blood cells (called lymphocytes) are found in the body. [NIH]

Ciliary: Inflammation or infection of the glands of the margins of the eyelids. [NIH]

CIS: Cancer Information Service. The CIS is the National Cancer Institute's link to the public, interpreting and explaining research findings in a clear and understandable manner, and providing personalized responses to specific questions about cancer. Access the CIS by calling 1-800-4-CANCER, or by using the Web site at http://cis.nci.nih.gov. [NIH]

Claudication: Limping or lameness. [EU]

Clinical study: A research study in which patients receive treatment in a clinic or other medical facility. Reports of clinical studies can contain results for single patients (case reports) or many patients (case series or clinical trials). [NIH]

Clinical trial: A research study that tests how well new medical treatments or other interventions work in people. Each study is designed to test new methods of screening, prevention, diagnosis, or treatment of a disease. [NIH]

Cloning: The production of a number of genetically identical individuals; in genetic engineering, a process for the efficient replication of a great number of identical DNA molecules. [NIH]

Colitis: Inflammation of the colon. [NIH]

Collagen: A polypeptide substance comprising about one third of the total protein in mammalian organisms. It is the main constituent of skin, connective tissue, and the organic substance of bones and teeth. Different forms of collagen are produced in the body but all consist of three alpha-polypeptide chains arranged in a triple helix. Collagen is differentiated from other fibrous proteins, such as elastin, by the content of proline, hydroxyproline, and hydroxylysine; by the absence of tryptophan; and particularly by the high content of polar groups which are responsible for its swelling properties. [NIH]

Colon: The long, coiled, tubelike organ that removes water from digested food. The remaining material, solid waste called stool, moves through the colon to the rectum and leaves the body through the anus. [NIH]

Complement: A term originally used to refer to the heat-labile factor in serum that causes immune cytolysis, the lysis of antibody-coated cells, and now referring to the entire functionally related system comprising at least 20 distinct serum proteins that is the effector not only of immune cytolysis but also of other biologic functions. Complement activation occurs by two different sequences, the classic and alternative pathways. The proteins of the classic pathway are termed 'components of complement' and are designated by the symbols C1 through C9. C1 is a calcium-dependent complex of three distinct proteins C1q, C1r and C1s. The proteins of the alternative pathway (collectively referred to as the properdin system) and complement regulatory proteins are known by semisystematic or trivial names. Fragments resulting from proteolytic cleavage of complement proteins are designated with lower-case letter suffixes, e.g., C3a. Inactivated fragments may be designated with the suffix 'i', e.g. C3bi. Activated components or complexes with biological activity are designated by a bar over the symbol e.g. C1 or C4b,2a. The classic pathway is activated by the binding of C1 to classic pathway activators, primarily antigen-antibody complexes containing IgM, IgG1, IgG3; C1q binds to a single IgM molecule or two adjacent IgG molecules. The alternative pathway can be activated by IgA immune complexes and also by nonimmunologic materials including bacterial endotoxins, microbial polysaccharides, and cell walls. Activation of the classic pathway triggers an enzymatic cascade involving C1, C4, C2 and C3; activation of the alternative pathway triggers a cascade involving C3 and factors B, D and P. Both result in the cleavage of C5 and the formation of the membrane attack complex. Complement activation also results in the formation of many biologically active complement fragments that act as anaphylatoxins, opsonins, or chemotactic factors. [EU]

Complementary and alternative medicine: CAM. Forms of treatment that are used in addition to (complementary) or instead of (alternative) standard treatments. These practices are not considered standard medical approaches. CAM includes dietary supplements, megadose vitamins, herbal preparations, special teas, massage therapy, magnet therapy, spiritual healing, and meditation. [NIH]

Complementary medicine: Practices not generally recognized by the medical community as standard or conventional medical approaches and used to enhance or complement the standard treatments. Complementary medicine includes the taking of dietary supplements, megadose vitamins, and herbal preparations; the drinking of special teas; and practices such as massage therapy, magnet therapy, spiritual healing, and meditation. [NIH]

Computational Biology: A field of biology concerned with the development of techniques for the collection and manipulation of biological data, and the use of such data to make biological discoveries or predictions. This field encompasses all computational methods and theories applicable to molecular biology and areas of computer-based techniques for solving biological problems including manipulation of models and datasets. [NIH]

Cones: One type of specialized light-sensitive cells (photoreceptors) in the retina that provide sharp central vision and color vision. [NIH]

Congestion: Excessive or abnormal accumulation of blood in a part. [EU]

Conjunctiva: The mucous membrane that lines the inner surface of the eyelids and the anterior part of the sclera. [NIH]

Conjunctivitis: Inflammation of the conjunctiva, generally consisting of conjunctival hyperaemia associated with a discharge. [EU]

Connective Tissue: Tissue that supports and binds other tissues. It consists of connective tissue cells embedded in a large amount of extracellular matrix. [NIH]

Connective Tissue: Tissue that supports and binds other tissues. It consists of connective tissue cells embedded in a large amount of extracellular matrix. [NIH]

Consciousness: Sense of awareness of self and of the environment. [NIH]

Constitutional: 1. Affecting the whole constitution of the body; not local. 2. Pertaining to the constitution. [EU]

Constriction: The act of constricting. [NIH]

Contamination: The soiling or pollution by inferior material, as by the introduction of organisms into a wound, or sewage into a stream. [EU]

Contraindications: Any factor or sign that it is unwise to pursue a certain kind of action or treatment, e. g. giving a general anesthetic to a person with pneumonia. [NIH]

Contralateral: Having to do with the opposite side of the body. [NIH]

Contrast medium: A substance that is introduced into or around a structure and, because of the difference in absorption of x-rays by the contrast medium and the surrounding tissues, allows radiographic visualization of the structure. [EU]

Cornea: The transparent part of the eye that covers the iris and the pupil and allows light to enter the inside. [NIH]

Coronary: Encircling in the manner of a crown; a term applied to vessels; nerves, ligaments, etc. The term usually denotes the arteries that supply the heart muscle and, by extension, a pathologic involvement of them. [EU]

Coronary heart disease: A type of heart disease caused by narrowing of the coronary arteries that feed the heart, which needs a constant supply of oxygen and nutrients carried by the blood in the coronary arteries. When the coronary arteries become narrowed or clogged by fat and cholesterol deposits and cannot supply enough blood to the heart, CHD results. [NIH]

Coronary Thrombosis: Presence of a thrombus in a coronary artery, often causing a myocardial infarction. [NIH]

Cortex: The outer layer of an organ or other body structure, as distinguished from the internal substance. [EU]

Corticosteroid: Any of the steroids elaborated by the adrenal cortex (excluding the sex hormones of adrenal origin) in response to the release of corticotrophin (adrenocorticotropic hormone) by the pituitary gland, to any of the synthetic equivalents of these steroids, or to angiotensin II. They are divided, according to their predominant biological activity, into three major groups: glucocorticoids, chiefly influencing carbohydrate, fat, and protein metabolism; mineralocorticoids, affecting the regulation of electrolyte and water balance; and C19 androgens. Some corticosteroids exhibit both types of activity in varying degrees, and others exert only one type of effect. The corticosteroids are used clinically for hormonal replacement therapy, for suppression of ACTH secretion by the anterior pituitary, as antineoplastic, antiallergic, and anti-inflammatory agents, and to suppress the immune response. Called also adrenocortical hormone and corticoid. [EU]

Cortisone: A natural steroid hormone produced in the adrenal gland. It can also be made in the laboratory. Cortisone reduces swelling and can suppress immune responses. [NIH]

Cranial: Pertaining to the cranium, or to the anterior (in animals) or superior (in humans) end of the body. [EU]

Craniocerebral Trauma: Traumatic injuries involving the cranium and intracranial structures (i.e., brain; cranial nerves; meninges; and other structures). Injuries may be classified by whether or not the skull is penetrated (i.e., penetrating vs. nonpenetrating) or whether there is an associated hemorrhage. [NIH]

Cutaneous: Having to do with the skin. [NIH]

Cyclic: Pertaining to or occurring in a cycle or cycles; the term is applied to chemical compounds that contain a ring of atoms in the nucleus. [EU]

Cytokine: Small but highly potent protein that modulates the activity of many cell types, including T and B cells. [NIH]

Cytoplasm: The protoplasm of a cell exclusive of that of the nucleus; it consists of a continuous aqueous solution (cytosol) and the organelles and inclusions suspended in it (phaneroplasm), and is the site of most of the chemical activities of the cell. [EU]

Degenerative: Undergoing degeneration : tending to degenerate; having the character of or involving degeneration; causing or tending to cause degeneration. [EU]

Dementia: An acquired organic mental disorder with loss of intellectual abilities of sufficient severity to interfere with social or occupational functioning. The dysfunction is multifaceted and involves memory, behavior, personality, judgment, attention, spatial relations, language, abstract thought, and other executive functions. The intellectual decline is usually progressive, and initially spares the level of consciousness. [NIH]

Denaturation: Rupture of the hydrogen bonds by heating a DNA solution and then cooling it rapidly causes the two complementary strands to separate. [NIH]

Dendrites: Extensions of the nerve cell body. They are short and branched and receive stimuli from other neurons. [NIH]

Dendritic: 1. Branched like a tree. 2. Pertaining to or possessing dendrites. [EU]

Dendritic cell: A special type of antigen-presenting cell (APC) that activates T lymphocytes. [NIH]

Density: The logarithm to the base 10 of the opacity of an exposed and processed film. [NIH]

Dentists: Individuals licensed to practice dentistry. [NIH]

Dermal: Pertaining to or coming from the skin. [NIH]

Dermatitis: Any inflammation of the skin. [NIH]

Dermatosis: Any skin disease, especially one not characterized by inflammation. [EU]

Dermis: A layer of vascular connective tissue underneath the epidermis. The surface of the dermis contains sensitive papillae. Embedded in or beneath the dermis are sweat glands, hair follicles, and sebaceous glands. [NIH]

Diagnostic procedure: A method used to identify a disease. [NIH]

Diaphragm: The musculofibrous partition that separates the thoracic cavity from the abdominal cavity. Contraction of the diaphragm increases the volume of the thoracic cavity aiding inspiration. [NIH]

Digestion: The process of breakdown of food for metabolism and use by the body. [NIH]

Digestive tract: The organs through which food passes when food is eaten. These organs are the mouth, esophagus, stomach, small and large intestines, and rectum. [NIH]

Direct: 1. Straight; in a straight line. 2. Performed immediately and without the intervention of subsidiary means. [EU]

Discrete: Made up of separate parts or characterized by lesions which do not become blended; not running together; separate. [NIH]

Dissection: Cutting up of an organism for study. [NIH]

Distal: Remote; farther from any point of reference; opposed to proximal. In dentistry, used to designate a position on the dental arch farther from the median line of the jaw. [EU]

Dorsal: 1. Pertaining to the back or to any dorsum. 2. Denoting a position more toward the back surface than some other object of reference; same as posterior in human anatomy; superior in the anatomy of quadrupeds. [EU]

Double-blind: Pertaining to a clinical trial or other experiment in which neither the subject nor the person administering treatment knows which treatment any particular subject is receiving. [EU]

Double-blinded: A clinical trial in which neither the medical staff nor the person knows which of several possible therapies the person is receiving. [NIH]

Drug Tolerance: Progressive diminution of the susceptibility of a human or animal to the effects of a drug, resulting from its continued administration. It should be differentiated from drug resistance wherein an organism, disease, or tissue fails to respond to the intended effectiveness of a chemical or drug. It should also be differentiated from maximum tolerated dose and no-observed-adverse-effect level. [NIH]

Duct: A tube through which body fluids pass. [NIH]

Edema: Excessive amount of watery fluid accumulated in the intercellular spaces, most commonly present in subcutaneous tissue. [NIH]

Effector: It is often an enzyme that converts an inactive precursor molecule into an active second messenger. [NIH]

Effector cell: A cell that performs a specific function in response to a stimulus; usually used to describe cells in the immune system. [NIH]

Elastin: The protein that gives flexibility to tissues. [NIH]

Elective: Subject to the choice or decision of the patient or physician; applied to procedures that are advantageous to the patient but not urgent. [EU]

Electrolyte: A substance that dissociates into ions when fused or in solution, and thus becomes capable of conducting electricity; an ionic solute. [EU]

Embolus: Bit of foreign matter which enters the blood stream at one point and is carried until it is lodged or impacted in an artery and obstructs it. It may be a blood clot, an air bubble, fat or other tissue, or clumps of bacteria. [NIH]

Endothelium: A layer of epithelium that lines the heart, blood vessels (endothelium, vascular), lymph vessels (endothelium, lymphatic), and the serous cavities of the body. [NIH]

Endothelium-derived: Small molecule that diffuses to the adjacent muscle layer and relaxes it. [NIH]

Environmental Health: The science of controlling or modifying those conditions, influences, or forces surrounding man which relate to promoting, establishing, and maintaining health. [NIH]

Enzymatic: Phase where enzyme cuts the precursor protein. [NIH]

Enzyme: A protein that speeds up chemical reactions in the body. [NIH]

Epidermal: Pertaining to or resembling epidermis. Called also epidermic or epidermoid. [EU]

Epidermis: Nonvascular layer of the skin. It is made up, from within outward, of five layers: 1) basal layer (stratum basale epidermidis); 2) spinous layer (stratum spinosum epidermidis); 3) granular layer (stratum granulosum epidermidis); 4) clear layer (stratum lucidum epidermidis); and 5) horny layer (stratum corneum epidermidis). [NIH]

Epidermoid carcinoma: A type of cancer in which the cells are flat and look like fish scales. Also called squamous cell carcinoma. [NIH]

Epithelium: One or more layers of epithelial cells, supported by the basal lamina, which covers the inner or outer surfaces of the body. [NIH]

Erythema: Redness of the skin produced by congestion of the capillaries. This condition may result from a variety of causes. [NIH]

Erythema Multiforme: A skin and mucous membrane disease characterized by an eruption of macules, papules, nodules, vesicles, and/or bullae with characteristic "bull's-eye" lesions usually occurring on the dorsal aspect of the hands and forearms. [NIH]

Extensor: A muscle whose contraction tends to straighten a limb; the antagonist of a flexor. [NIH]

Extracellular: Outside a cell or cells. [EU]

Extracellular Matrix: A meshwork-like substance found within the extracellular space and in association with the basement membrane of the cell surface. It promotes cellular proliferation and provides a supporting structure to which cells or cell lysates in culture dishes adhere. [NIH]

Extracellular Matrix Proteins: Macromolecular organic compounds that contain carbon, hydrogen, oxygen, nitrogen, and usually, sulfur. These macromolecules (proteins) form an intricate meshwork in which cells are embedded to construct tissues. Variations in the relative types of macromolecules and their organization determine the type of extracellular matrix, each adapted to the functional requirements of the tissue. The two main classes of macromolecules that form the extracellular matrix are: glycosaminoglycans, usually linked to proteins (proteoglycans), and fibrous proteins (e.g., collagen, elastin, fibronectins and laminin). [NIH]

Extravasation: A discharge or escape, as of blood, from a vessel into the tissues. [EU]

Extremity: A limb; an arm or leg (membrum); sometimes applied specifically to a hand or foot. [EU]

Facial: Of or pertaining to the face. [EU]

Facial Nerve: The 7th cranial nerve. The facial nerve has two parts, the larger motor root which may be called the facial nerve proper, and the smaller intermediate or sensory root. Together they provide efferent innervation to the muscles of facial expression and to the lacrimal and salivary glands, and convey afferent information for taste from the anterior two-thirds of the tongue and for touch from the external ear. [NIH]

Family Planning: Programs or services designed to assist the family in controlling reproduction by either improving or diminishing fertility. [NIH]

Fat: Total lipids including phospholipids. [NIH]

Febrile: Pertaining to or characterized by fever. [EU]

Femoral: Pertaining to the femur, or to the thigh. [EU]

Femur: The longest and largest bone of the skeleton, it is situated between the hip and the knee. [NIH]

Fetus: The developing offspring from 7 to 8 weeks after conception until birth. [NIH]

Fibrinolysis: The natural enzymatic dissolution of fibrin. [NIH]

Fibrosis: Any pathological condition where fibrous connective tissue invades any organ, usually as a consequence of inflammation or other injury. [NIH]

Flexor: Muscles which flex a joint. [NIH]

Gamma-interferon: Interferon produced by T-lymphocytes in response to various mitogens and antigens. Gamma interferon appears to have potent antineoplastic, immunoregulatory and antiviral activity. [NIH]

Ganglion: 1. A knot, or knotlike mass. 2. A general term for a group of nerve cell bodies located outside the central nervous system; occasionally applied to certain nuclear groups within the brain or spinal cord, e.g. basal ganglia. 3. A benign cystic tumour occurring on a aponeurosis or tendon, as in the wrist or dorsum of the foot; it consists of a thin fibrous capsule enclosing a clear mucinous fluid. [EU]

Gangrene: Death and putrefaction of tissue usually due to a loss of blood supply. [NIH]

Gas: Air that comes from normal breakdown of food. The gases are passed out of the body through the rectum (flatus) or the mouth (burp). [NIH]

Gastrin: A hormone released after eating. Gastrin causes the stomach to produce more acid. [NIH]

Gene: The functional and physical unit of heredity passed from parent to offspring. Genes are pieces of DNA, and most genes contain the information for making a specific protein. [NIH]

Gene Expression: The phenotypic manifestation of a gene or genes by the processes of gene action. [NIH]

Gene Expression Profiling: The determination of the pattern of genes expressed i.e., transcribed, under specific circumstances or in a specific cell. [NIH]

Genetic testing: Analyzing DNA to look for a genetic alteration that may indicate an increased risk for developing a specific disease or disorder. [NIH]

Genital: Pertaining to the genitalia. [EU]

Giant Cells: Multinucleated masses produced by the fusion of many cells; often associated with viral infections. In AIDS, they are induced when the envelope glycoprotein of the HIV virus binds to the CD4 antigen of uninfected neighboring T4 cells. The resulting syncytium leads to cell death and thus may account for the cytopathic effect of the virus. [NIH]

Gingival Hyperplasia: A pathological increase in the depth of the gingival crevice surrounding a tooth at the gum margin. [NIH]

Gingivitis: Inflammation of the gingivae. Gingivitis associated with bony changes is referred to as periodontitis. Called also oulitis and ulitis. [EU]

Gland: An organ that produces and releases one or more substances for use in the body. Some glands produce fluids that affect tissues or organs. Others produce hormones or participate in blood production. [NIH]

Glomerular: Pertaining to or of the nature of a glomerulus, especially a renal glomerulus. [EU]

Glucocorticoid: A compound that belongs to the family of compounds called corticosteroids (steroids). Glucocorticoids affect metabolism and have anti-inflammatory and immunosuppressive effects. They may be naturally produced (hormones) or synthetic (drugs). [NIH]

Glucose: D-Glucose. A primary source of energy for living organisms. It is naturally occurring and is found in fruits and other parts of plants in its free state. It is used therapeutically in fluid and nutrient replacement. [NIH]

Glycoprotein: A protein that has sugar molecules attached to it. [NIH]

Gonadal: Pertaining to a gonad. [EU]

Governing Board: The group in which legal authority is vested for the control of health-related institutions and organizations. [NIH]

Graft: Healthy skin, bone, or other tissue taken from one part of the body and used to replace diseased or injured tissue removed from another part of the body. [NIH]

Graft-versus-host disease: GVHD. A reaction of donated bone marrow or peripheral stem cells against a person's tissue. [NIH]

Granuloma: A relatively small nodular inflammatory lesion containing grouped mononuclear phagocytes, caused by infectious and noninfectious agents. [NIH]

Guanylate Cyclase: An enzyme that catalyzes the conversion of GTP to 3',5'-cyclic GMP and pyrophosphate. It also acts on ITP and dGTP. (From Enzyme Nomenclature, 1992) EC 4.6.1.2. [NIH]

Haematuria: Blood in the urine. [EU]

Halitosis: An offensive, foul breath odor resulting from a variety of causes such as poor oral hygiene, dental or oral infections, or the ingestion of certain foods. [NIH]

Hantavirus: A genus of the family Bunyaviridae causing Hantavirus infections, first identified during the Korean war. Infection is found primarily in rodents and humans. Transmission does not appear to involve arthropods. The genus has one recognized group (Hantaan group) consisting of several species including Dobrava-Belgrade virus, Seoul virus, Prospect Hill virus, Puumala virus, Thottapalayam virus, and Hantaan virus, the type species. [NIH]

Hantavirus Infections: Infections with viruses of the genus Hantavirus. This is associated with at least four clinical syndromes: hemorrhagic fever with renal syndrome caused by viruses of the Hantaan group; a milder form of HFRS caused by Seoul and related viruses; nephropathia epidemica caused by Puumala and related viruses; and hantavirus pulmonary syndrome caused by Muerto Canyon virus. [NIH]

Hantavirus Pulmonary Syndrome: Acute respiratory illness in humans caused by the Muerto Canyon virus whose primary rodent reservoir is the deer mouse Peromyscus maniculatus. First identified in the southwestern United States, this syndrome is characterized most commonly by fever, myalgias, headache, cough, and rapid respiratory failure. [NIH]

Headache: Pain in the cranial region that may occur as an isolated and benign symptom or as a manifestation of a wide variety of conditions including subarachnoid hemorrhage; craniocerebral trauma; central nervous system infections; intracranial hypertension; and other disorders. In general, recurrent headaches that are not associated with a primary disease process are referred to as headache disorders (e.g., migraine). [NIH]

Headache Disorders: Common conditions characterized by persistent or recurrent headaches. Headache syndrome classification systems may be based on etiology (e.g., vascular headache, post-traumatic headaches, etc.), temporal pattern (e.g., cluster headache, paroxysmal hemicrania, etc.), and precipitating factors (e.g., cough headache). [NIH]

Heart attack: A seizure of weak or abnormal functioning of the heart. [NIH]

Heart failure: Loss of pumping ability by the heart, often accompanied by fatigue, breathlessness, and excess fluid accumulation in body tissues. [NIH]

Hematoma: An extravasation of blood localized in an organ, space, or tissue. [NIH]

Hemorrhage: Bleeding or escape of blood from a vessel. [NIH]

Hepatitis: Inflammation of the liver and liver disease involving degenerative or necrotic alterations of hepatocytes. [NIH]

Hepatitis A: Hepatitis caused by hepatovirus. It can be transmitted through fecal contamination of food or water. [NIH]

Hepatocytes: The main structural component of the liver. They are specialized epithelial cells that are organized into interconnected plates called lobules. [NIH]

Hepatovirus: A genus of Picornaviridae causing infectious hepatitis naturally in humans and experimentally in other primates. It is transmitted through fecal contamination of food or water. [NIH]

Heredity: 1. The genetic transmission of a particular quality or trait from parent to offspring. 2. The genetic constitution of an individual. [EU]

Herpes: Any inflammatory skin disease caused by a herpesvirus and characterized by the formation of clusters of small vesicles. When used alone, the term may refer to herpes simplex or to herpes zoster. [EU]

Herpes virus: A member of the herpes family of viruses. [NIH]

Herpes Zoster: Acute vesicular inflammation. [NIH]

Heterogeneity: The property of one or more samples or populations which implies that they are not identical in respect of some or all of their parameters, e. g. heterogeneity of variance. [NIH]

Histology: The study of tissues and cells under a microscope. [NIH]

Homologous: Corresponding in structure, position, origin, etc., as (a) the feathers of a bird and the scales of a fish, (b) antigen and its specific antibody, (c) allelic chromosomes. [EU]

Hormonal: Pertaining to or of the nature of a hormone. [EU]

Hormone: A substance in the body that regulates certain organs. Hormones such as gastrin help in breaking down food. Some hormones come from cells in the stomach and small intestine. [NIH]

Hyperaemia: An excess of blood in a part; engorgement. [EU]

Hyperplasia: An increase in the number of cells in a tissue or organ, not due to tumor formation. It differs from hypertrophy, which is an increase in bulk without an increase in the number of cells. [NIH]

Hypersensitivity: Altered reactivity to an antigen, which can result in pathologic reactions upon subsequent exposure to that particular antigen. [NIH]

Hypertension: Persistently high arterial blood pressure. Currently accepted threshold levels are 140 mm Hg systolic and 90 mm Hg diastolic pressure. [NIH]

Immune response: The activity of the immune system against foreign substances (antigens). [NIH]

Immune system: The organs, cells, and molecules responsible for the recognition and disposal of foreign ("non-self") material which enters the body. [NIH]

Immune Tolerance: The specific failure of a normally responsive individual to make an immune response to a known antigen. It results from previous contact with the antigen by an immunologically immature individual (fetus or neonate) or by an adult exposed to extreme high-dose or low-dose antigen, or by exposure to radiation, antimetabolites, antilymphocytic serum, etc. [NIH]

Immunoglobulin: A protein that acts as an antibody. [NIH]

Immunology: The study of the body's immune system. [NIH]

Immunosuppressant: An agent capable of suppressing immune responses. [EU]

Immunosuppressive: Describes the ability to lower immune system responses. [NIH]

Infarction: A pathological process consisting of a sudden insufficient blood supply to an area, which results in necrosis of that area. It is usually caused by a thrombus, an embolus, or a vascular torsion. [NIH]

Infection: 1. Invasion and multiplication of microorganisms in body tissues, which may be clinically unapparent or result in local cellular injury due to competitive metabolism, toxins, intracellular replication, or antigen-antibody response. The infection may remain localized, subclinical, and temporary if the body's defensive mechanisms are effective. A local infection may persist and spread by extension to become an acute, subacute, or chronic clinical infection or disease state. A local infection may also become systemic when the microorganisms gain access to the lymphatic or vascular system. 2. An infectious disease. [EU]

Infiltration: The diffusion or accumulation in a tissue or cells of substances not normal to it or in amounts of the normal. Also, the material so accumulated. [EU]

Inflammation: A pathological process characterized by injury or destruction of tissues caused by a variety of cytologic and chemical reactions. It is usually manifested by typical signs of pain, heat, redness, swelling, and loss of function. [NIH]

Inflammatory bowel disease: A general term that refers to the inflammation of the colon and rectum. Inflammatory bowel disease includes ulcerative colitis and Crohn's disease. [NIH]

Ingestion: Taking into the body by mouth [NIH]

Initiation: Mutation induced by a chemical reactive substance causing cell changes; being a step in a carcinogenic process. [NIH]

Innervation: 1. The distribution or supply of nerves to a part. 2. The supply of nervous energy or of nerve stimulus sent to a part. [EU]

Intercellular Adhesion Molecule-1: A cell-surface ligand with a role in leukocyte adhesion and inflammation. Its production is induced by gamma-interferon and it is required for neutrophil migration into inflamed tissue. [NIH]

Interstitial: Pertaining to or situated between parts or in the interspaces of a tissue. [EU]

Intervertebral: Situated between two contiguous vertebrae. [EU]

Intestine: A long, tube-shaped organ in the abdomen that completes the process of digestion. There is both a large intestine and a small intestine. Also called the bowel. [NIH]

Intracellular: Inside a cell. [NIH]

Intravenous: IV. Into a vein. [NIH]

Invasive: 1. Having the quality of invasiveness. 2. Involving puncture or incision of the skin or insertion of an instrument or foreign material into the body; said of diagnostic techniques. [EU]

Ipsilateral: Having to do with the same side of the body. [NIH]

Ischemia: Deficiency of blood in a part, due to functional constriction or actual obstruction of a blood vessel. [EU]

Kb: A measure of the length of DNA fragments, 1 Kb = 1000 base pairs. The largest DNA fragments are up to 50 kilobases long. [NIH]

Keratoconjunctivitis: Simultaneous inflammation of the cornea and conjunctiva. [NIH]

Keratoconjunctivitis Sicca: Drying and inflammation of the conjunctiva as a result of insufficient lacrimal secretion. When found in association with xerostomia and polyarthritis, it is called Sjogren's syndrome. [NIH]

Keratosis: Any horny growth such as a wart or callus. [NIH]

Lacrimal: Pertaining to the tears. [EU]

Lectin: A complex molecule that has both protein and sugars. Lectins are able to bind to the outside of a cell and cause biochemical changes in it. Lectins are made by both animals and plants. [NIH]

Lesion: An area of abnormal tissue change. [NIH]

Leucocyte: All the white cells of the blood and their precursors (myeloid cell series, lymphoid cell series) but commonly used to indicate granulocytes exclusive of lymphocytes. [NIH]

Leukaemia: An acute or chronic disease of unknown cause in man and other warm-blooded animals that involves the blood-forming organs, is characterized by an abnormal increase in the number of leucocytes in the tissues of the body with or without a corresponding increase of those in the circulating blood, and is classified according of the type leucocyte most prominently involved. [EU]

Leukemia: Cancer of blood-forming tissue. [NIH]

Leukocytes: White blood cells. These include granular leukocytes (basophils, eosinophils, and neutrophils) as well as non-granular leukocytes (lymphocytes and monocytes). [NIH]

Leukoplakia: A white patch that may develop on mucous membranes such as the cheek, gums, or tongue and may become cancerous. [NIH]

Lichen Planus: An inflammatory, pruritic disease of the skin and mucous membranes, which can be either generalized or localized. It is characterized by distinctive purplish, flat-topped papules having a predilection for the trunk and flexor surfaces. The lesions may be discrete or coalesce to form plaques. Histologically, there is a "saw-tooth" pattern of epidermal hyperplasia and vacuolar alteration of the basal layer of the epidermis along with an intense upper dermal inflammatory infiltrate composed predominantly of T-cells. Etiology is unknown. [NIH]

Life cycle: The successive stages through which an organism passes from fertilized ovum or spore to the fertilized ovum or spore of the next generation. [NIH]

Ligaments: Shiny, flexible bands of fibrous tissue connecting together articular extremities of bones. They are pliant, tough, and inextensile. [NIH]

Lip: Either of the two fleshy, full-blooded margins of the mouth. [NIH]

Liver: A large, glandular organ located in the upper abdomen. The liver cleanses the blood and aids in digestion by secreting bile. [NIH]

Localized: Cancer which has not metastasized yet. [NIH]

Lumbar: Pertaining to the loins, the part of the back between the thorax and the pelvis. [EU]

Lupus: A form of cutaneous tuberculosis. It is seen predominantly in women and typically involves the nasal, buccal, and conjunctival mucosa. [NIH]

Lymph: The almost colorless fluid that travels through the lymphatic system and carries cells that help fight infection and disease. [NIH]

Lymph node: A rounded mass of lymphatic tissue that is surrounded by a capsule of connective tissue. Also known as a lymph gland. Lymph nodes are spread out along lymphatic vessels and contain many lymphocytes, which filter the lymphatic fluid (lymph). [NIH]

Lymphatic: The tissues and organs, including the bone marrow, spleen, thymus, and lymph nodes, that produce and store cells that fight infection and disease. [NIH]

Lymphocyte: A white blood cell. Lymphocytes have a number of roles in the immune system, including the production of antibodies and other substances that fight infection and diseases. [NIH]

Lymphocytic: Referring to lymphocytes, a type of white blood cell. [NIH]

Lymphoid: Referring to lymphocytes, a type of white blood cell. Also refers to tissue in which lymphocytes develop. [NIH]

Macrophage: A type of white blood cell that surrounds and kills microorganisms, removes dead cells, and stimulates the action of other immune system cells. [NIH]

Magnetic Resonance Imaging: Non-invasive method of demonstrating internal anatomy based on the principle that atomic nuclei in a strong magnetic field absorb pulses of radiofrequency energy and emit them as radiowaves which can be reconstructed into computerized images. The concept includes proton spin tomographic techniques. [NIH]

Malaise: A vague feeling of bodily discomfort. [EU]

Malignant: Cancerous; a growth with a tendency to invade and destroy nearby tissue and spread to other parts of the body. [NIH]

Malignant tumor: A tumor capable of metastasizing. [NIH]

Masseter Muscle: A masticatory muscle whose action is closing the jaws. [NIH]

Matrix metalloproteinase: A member of a group of enzymes that can break down proteins, such as collagen, that are normally found in the spaces between cells in tissues (i.e., extracellular matrix proteins). Because these enzymes need zinc or calcium atoms to work properly, they are called metalloproteinases. Matrix metalloproteinases are involved in wound healing, angiogenesis, and tumor cell metastasis. [NIH]

Maxillary: Pertaining to the maxilla : the irregularly shaped bone that with its fellow forms the upper jaw. [EU]

Maxillary Artery: A branch of the external carotid artery which distributes to the deep structures of the face (internal maxillary) and to the side of the face and nose (external maxillary). [NIH]

Median Nerve: A major nerve of the upper extremity. In humans, the fibers of the median nerve originate in the lower cervical and upper thoracic spinal cord (usually C6 to T1), travel via the brachial plexus, and supply sensory and motor innervation to parts of the forearm and hand. [NIH]

Medical Staff: Professional medical personnel who provide care to patients in an organized facility, institution or agency. [NIH]

MEDLINE: An online database of MEDLARS, the computerized bibliographic Medical Literature Analysis and Retrieval System of the National Library of Medicine. [NIH]

Membrane: A very thin layer of tissue that covers a surface. [NIH]

Memory: Complex mental function having four distinct phases: (1) memorizing or learning, (2) retention, (3) recall, and (4) recognition. Clinically, it is usually subdivided into immediate, recent, and remote memory. [NIH]

Meninges: The three membranes that cover and protect the brain and spinal cord. [NIH]

Mental: Pertaining to the mind; psychic. 2. (L. mentum chin) pertaining to the chin. [EU]

Metastasis: The spread of cancer from one part of the body to another. Tumors formed from cells that have spread are called "secondary tumors" and contain cells that are like those in the original (primary) tumor. The plural is metastases. [NIH]

Methotrexate: An antineoplastic antimetabolite with immunosuppressant properties. It is an inhibitor of dihydrofolate reductase and prevents the formation of tetrahydrofolate, necessary for synthesis of thymidylate, an essential component of DNA. [NIH]

Methylprednisolone: (6 alpha,11 beta)-11,17,21-Trihydroxy-6-methylpregna-1,4-diene-3,2-dione. A prednisolone derivative which has pharmacological actions similar to prednisolone. [NIH]

MI: Myocardial infarction. Gross necrosis of the myocardium as a result of interruption of the blood supply to the area; it is almost always caused by atherosclerosis of the coronary arteries, upon which coronary thrombosis is usually superimposed. [NIH]

Mice Minute Virus: The type species of parvovirus prevalent in mouse colonies and found as a contaminant of many transplanted tumors or leukemias. [NIH]

Microbiology: The study of microorganisms such as fungi, bacteria, algae, archaea, and viruses. [NIH]

Middle Cerebral Artery: The largest and most complex of the cerebral arteries. Branches of the middle cerebral artery supply the insular region, motor and premotor areas, and large regions of the association cortex. [NIH]

Migration: The systematic movement of genes between populations of the same species, geographic race, or variety. [NIH]

Mineralocorticoids: A group of corticosteroids primarily associated with the regulation of water and electrolyte balance. This is accomplished through the effect on ion transport in renal tubules, resulting in retention of sodium and loss of potassium. Mineralocorticoid secretion is itself regulated by plasma volume, serum potassium, and angiotensin II. [NIH]

Mitochondrial Swelling: Increase in volume of mitochondria due to an influx of fluid; it occurs in hypotonic solutions due to osmotic pressure and in isotonic solutions as a result of altered permeability of the membranes of respiring mitochondria. [NIH]

Modification: A change in an organism, or in a process in an organism, that is acquired from its own activity or environment. [NIH]

Molecular: Of, pertaining to, or composed of molecules : a very small mass of matter. [EU]

Molecule: A chemical made up of two or more atoms. The atoms in a molecule can be the same (an oxygen molecule has two oxygen atoms) or different (a water molecule has two hydrogen atoms and one oxygen atom). Biological molecules, such as proteins and DNA, can be made up of many thousands of atoms. [NIH]

Monoclonal: An antibody produced by culturing a single type of cell. It therefore consists of a single species of immunoglobulin molecules. [NIH]

Monocular: Diplopia identified with one eye only; it may be induced with a double prism, or it may occur either as a result of double imagery due to an optical defect in the eye, or as a result of simultaneous use of normal and anomalous retinal correspondence. [NIH]

Monocytes: Large, phagocytic mononuclear leukocytes produced in the vertebrate bone marrow and released into the blood; contain a large, oval or somewhat indented nucleus surrounded by voluminous cytoplasm and numerous organelles. [NIH]

Mononuclear: A cell with one nucleus. [NIH]

Monotherapy: A therapy which uses only one drug. [EU]

Motor nerve: An efferent nerve conveying an impulse that excites muscular contraction. [NIH]

Mucosa: A mucous membrane, or tunica mucosa. [EU]

Myasthenia: Muscular debility; any constitutional anomaly of muscle. [EU]

Myeloma: Cancer that arises in plasma cells, a type of white blood cell. [NIH]

Myocardial infarction: Gross necrosis of the myocardium as a result of interruption of the blood supply to the area; it is almost always caused by atherosclerosis of the coronary arteries, upon which coronary thrombosis is usually superimposed. [NIH]

Myocardium: The muscle tissue of the heart composed of striated, involuntary muscle known as cardiac muscle. [NIH]

Myositis: Inflammation of a voluntary muscle. [EU]

Necrosis: A pathological process caused by the progressive degradative action of enzymes that is generally associated with severe cellular trauma. It is characterized by mitochondrial swelling, nuclear flocculation, uncontrolled cell lysis, and ultimately cell death. [NIH]

Neoplasm: A new growth of benign or malignant tissue. [NIH]

Neoplastic: Pertaining to or like a neoplasm (= any new and abnormal growth); pertaining to neoplasia (= the formation of a neoplasm). [EU]

Nerve: A cordlike structure of nervous tissue that connects parts of the nervous system with other tissues of the body and conveys nervous impulses to, or away from, these tissues. [NIH]

Nervous System: The entire nerve apparatus composed of the brain, spinal cord, nerves and ganglia. [NIH]

Networks: Pertaining to a nerve or to the nerves, a meshlike structure of interlocking fibers or strands. [NIH]

Neuromuscular: Pertaining to muscles and nerves. [EU]

Neuromuscular Junction: The synapse between a neuron and a muscle. [NIH]

Neuropathy: A problem in any part of the nervous system except the brain and spinal cord. Neuropathies can be caused by infection, toxic substances, or disease. [NIH]

Neutrophil: A type of white blood cell. [NIH]

Nitric Oxide: A free radical gas produced endogenously by a variety of mammalian cells. It is synthesized from arginine by a complex reaction, catalyzed by nitric oxide synthase. Nitric oxide is endothelium-derived relaxing factor. It is released by the vascular endothelium and mediates the relaxation induced by some vasodilators such as acetylcholine and bradykinin. It also inhibits platelet aggregation, induces disaggregation of aggregated platelets, and inhibits platelet adhesion to the vascular endothelium. Nitric oxide activates cytosolic guanylate cyclase and thus elevates intracellular levels of cyclic GMP. [NIH]

Nitrogen: An element with the atomic symbol N, atomic number 7, and atomic weight 14. Nitrogen exists as a diatomic gas and makes up about 78% of the earth's atmosphere by volume. It is a constituent of proteins and nucleic acids and found in all living cells. [NIH]

Nuclear: A test of the structure, blood flow, and function of the kidneys. The doctor injects a mildly radioactive solution into an arm vein and uses x-rays to monitor its progress through the kidneys. [NIH]

Nuclei: A body of specialized protoplasm found in nearly all cells and containing the chromosomes. [NIH]

Nucleic acid: Either of two types of macromolecule (DNA or RNA) formed by polymerization of nucleotides. Nucleic acids are found in all living cells and contain the information (genetic code) for the transfer of genetic information from one generation to the next. [NIH]

Nucleus: A body of specialized protoplasm found in nearly all cells and containing the chromosomes. [NIH]

Occult: Obscure; concealed from observation, difficult to understand. [EU]

Ocular: 1. Of, pertaining to, or affecting the eye. 2. Eyepiece. [EU]

Oculomotor: Cranial nerve III. It originate from the lower ventral surface of the midbrain and is classified as a motor nerve. [NIH]

Oculomotor Nerve: The 3d cranial nerve. The oculomotor nerve sends motor fibers to the levator muscles of the eyelid and to the superior rectus, inferior rectus, and inferior oblique muscles of the eye. It also sends parasympathetic efferents (via the ciliary ganglion) to the muscles controlling pupillary constriction and accommodation. The motor fibers originate in the oculomotor nuclei of the midbrain. [NIH]

Oedema: The presence of abnormally large amounts of fluid in the intercellular tissue spaces of the body; usually applied to demonstrable accumulation of excessive fluid in the subcutaneous tissues. Edema may be localized, due to venous or lymphatic obstruction or to increased vascular permeability, or it may be systemic due to heart failure or renal disease. Collections of edema fluid are designated according to the site, e.g. ascites (peritoneal cavity), hydrothorax (pleural cavity), and hydropericardium (pericardial sac). Massive generalized edema is called anasarca. [EU]

Opacity: Degree of density (area most dense taken for reading). [NIH]

Ophthalmic: Pertaining to the eye. [EU]

Ophthalmic Artery: Artery originating from the internal carotid artery and distributing to the eye, orbit and adjacent facial structures. [NIH]

Ophthalmologic: Pertaining to ophthalmology (= the branch of medicine dealing with the eye). [EU]

Ophthalmology: A surgical specialty concerned with the structure and function of the eye and the medical and surgical treatment of its defects and diseases. [NIH]

Ophthalmoplegia: Paralysis of one or more of the ocular muscles due to disorders of the eye muscles, neuromuscular junction, supporting soft tissue, tendons, or innervation to the muscles. [NIH]

Opsin: A protein formed, together with retinene, by the chemical breakdown of meta-rhodopsin. [NIH]

Optic Chiasm: The X-shaped structure formed by the meeting of the two optic nerves. At the optic chiasm the fibers from the medial part of each retina cross to project to the other side of the brain while the lateral retinal fibers continue on the same side. As a result each half of the brain receives information about the contralateral visual field from both eyes. [NIH]

Optic Nerve: The 2nd cranial nerve. The optic nerve conveys visual information from the retina to the brain. The nerve carries the axons of the retinal ganglion cells which sort at the optic chiasm and continue via the optic tracts to the brain. The largest projection is to the lateral geniculate nuclei; other important targets include the superior colliculi and the suprachiasmatic nuclei. Though known as the second cranial nerve, it is considered part of the central nervous system. [NIH]

Oral Hygiene: The practice of personal hygiene of the mouth. It includes the maintenance of oral cleanliness, tissue tone, and general preservation of oral health. [NIH]

Organelles: Specific particles of membrane-bound organized living substances present in eukaryotic cells, such as the mitochondria; the golgi apparatus; endoplasmic reticulum; lysomomes; plastids; and vacuoles. [NIH]

Otitis: Inflammation of the ear, which may be marked by pain, fever, abnormalities of hearing, hearing loss, tinnitus, and vertigo. [EU]

Ovum: A female germ cell extruded from the ovary at ovulation. [NIH]

Palate: The structure that forms the roof of the mouth. It consists of the anterior hard palate and the posterior soft palate. [NIH]

Pallor: A clinical manifestation consisting of an unnatural paleness of the skin. [NIH]

Palsy: Disease of the peripheral nervous system occurring usually after many years of increased lead absorption. [NIH]

Paralysis: Loss of ability to move all or part of the body. [NIH]

Parasite: An animal or a plant that lives on or in an organism of another species and gets at least some of its nutrition from that other organism. [NIH]

Parasitic: Having to do with or being a parasite. A parasite is an animal or a plant that lives on or in an organism of another species and gets at least some of its nutrients from it. [NIH]

Parasitic Diseases: Infections or infestations with parasitic organisms. They are often contracted through contact with an intermediate vector, but may occur as the result of direct exposure. [NIH]

Parietal: 1. Of or pertaining to the walls of a cavity. 2. Pertaining to or located near the parietal bone, as the parietal lobe. [EU]

Parotid: The space that contains the parotid gland, the facial nerve, the external carotid artery, and the retromandibular vein. [NIH]

Parvovirus: A genus of the family Parvoviridae, subfamily Parvovirinae, infecting a variety of vertebrates including humans. Parvoviruses are responsible for a number of important diseases but also can be non-pathogenic in certain hosts. The type species is mice minute virus. [NIH]

Patch: A piece of material used to cover or protect a wound, an injured part, etc.: a patch over the eye. [NIH]

Pathogenesis: The cellular events and reactions that occur in the development of disease. [NIH]

Pathologic: 1. Indicative of or caused by a morbid condition. 2. Pertaining to pathology (= branch of medicine that treats the essential nature of the disease, especially the structural and functional changes in tissues and organs of the body caused by the disease). [EU]

Pelvis: The lower part of the abdomen, located between the hip bones. [NIH]

Percutaneous: Performed through the skin, as injection of radiopacque material in radiological examination, or the removal of tissue for biopsy accomplished by a needle. [EU]

Periodontitis: Inflammation of the periodontal membrane; also called periodontitis simplex. [NIH]

Perioral: Situated or occurring around the mouth. [EU]

Peripheral blood: Blood circulating throughout the body. [NIH]

Peripheral Nervous System: The nervous system outside of the brain and spinal cord. The peripheral nervous system has autonomic and somatic divisions. The autonomic nervous system includes the enteric, parasympathetic, and sympathetic subdivisions. The somatic nervous system includes the cranial and spinal nerves and their ganglia and the peripheral sensory receptors. [NIH]

Peripheral stem cells: Immature cells found circulating in the bloodstream. New blood cells develop from peripheral stem cells. [NIH]

Peritoneal: Having to do with the peritoneum (the tissue that lines the abdominal wall and covers most of the organs in the abdomen). [NIH]

Peritoneal Cavity: The space enclosed by the peritoneum. It is divided into two portions, the greater sac and the lesser sac or omental bursa, which lies behind the stomach. The two sacs are connected by the foramen of Winslow, or epiploic foramen. [NIH]

Pharmacologic: Pertaining to pharmacology or to the properties and reactions of drugs. [EU]

Phosphenes: Visual sensations arising from mechanical or electrical stimulation of the eyeball. [NIH]

Physiologic: Having to do with the functions of the body. When used in the phrase "physiologic age," it refers to an age assigned by general health, as opposed to calendar age. [NIH]

Pigment: A substance that gives color to tissue. Pigments are responsible for the color of skin, eyes, and hair. [NIH]

Pigmentation: Coloration or discoloration of a part by a pigment. [NIH]

Pilot study: The initial study examining a new method or treatment. [NIH]

Pituitary Gland: A small, unpaired gland situated in the sella turcica tissue. It is connected to the hypothalamus by a short stalk. [NIH]

Plants: Multicellular, eukaryotic life forms of the kingdom Plantae. They are characterized by a mainly photosynthetic mode of nutrition; essentially unlimited growth at localized regions of cell divisions (meristems); cellulose within cells providing rigidity; the absence of organs of locomotion; absense of nervous and sensory systems; and an alteration of haploid and diploid generations. [NIH]

Plasma: The clear, yellowish, fluid part of the blood that carries the blood cells. The proteins that form blood clots are in plasma. [NIH]

Plasma cells: A type of white blood cell that produces antibodies. [NIH]

Platelet Aggregation: The attachment of platelets to one another. This clumping together can be induced by a number of agents (e.g., thrombin, collagen) and is part of the mechanism leading to the formation of a thrombus. [NIH]

Platelets: A type of blood cell that helps prevent bleeding by causing blood clots to form. Also called thrombocytes. [NIH]

Pleura: The thin serous membrane enveloping the lungs and lining the thoracic cavity. [NIH]

Pleural: A circumscribed area of hyaline whorled fibrous tissue which appears on the surface of the parietal pleura, on the fibrous part of the diaphragm or on the pleura in the interlobar fissures. [NIH]

Pleural cavity: A space enclosed by the pleura (thin tissue covering the lungs and lining the interior wall of the chest cavity). It is bound by thin membranes. [NIH]

Pleural Effusion: Presence of fluid in the pleural cavity resulting from excessive transudation or exudation from the pleural surfaces. It is a sign of disease and not a diagnosis in itself. [NIH]

Pneumonia: Inflammation of the lungs. [NIH]

Polyarteritis Nodosa: A form of necrotizing vasculitis involving small- and medium-sized arteries. The signs and symptoms result from infarction and scarring of the affected organ system. [NIH]

Polyarthritis: An inflammation of several joints together. [EU]

Polymerase: An enzyme which catalyses the synthesis of DNA using a single DNA strand as a template. The polymerase copies the template in the 5'-3'direction provided that sufficient quantities of free nucleotides, dATP and dTTP are present. [NIH]

Polymerase Chain Reaction: In vitro method for producing large amounts of specific DNA or RNA fragments of defined length and sequence from small amounts of short oligonucleotide flanking sequences (primers). The essential steps include thermal denaturation of the double-stranded target molecules, annealing of the primers to their complementary sequences, and extension of the annealed primers by enzymatic synthesis with DNA polymerase. The reaction is efficient, specific, and extremely sensitive. Uses for the reaction include disease diagnosis, detection of difficult-to-isolate pathogens, mutation analysis, genetic testing, DNA sequencing, and analyzing evolutionary relationships. [NIH]

Polymorphism: The occurrence together of two or more distinct forms in the same population. [NIH]

Polymyalgia Rheumatica: A syndrome in the elderly characterized by proximal joint and muscle pain, high erythrocyte sedimentation rate, and a self-limiting course. Pain is usually accompanied by evidence of an inflammatory reaction. Women are affected twice as commonly as men and Caucasians more frequently than other groups. The condition is frequently associated with temporal arteritis and some theories pose the possibility that the two diseases arise from a single etiology or even that they are the same entity. [NIH]

Polysaccharide: A type of carbohydrate. It contains sugar molecules that are linked together chemically. [NIH]

Polytetrafluoroethylene: Homopolymer of tetrafluoroethylene. Nonflammable, tough, inert plastic tubing or sheeting; used to line vessels, insulate, protect or lubricate apparatus; also as filter, coating for surgical implants or as prosthetic material. Synonyms: Fluoroflex; Fluoroplast; Ftoroplast; Halon; Polyfene; PTFE; Tetron. [NIH]

Posterior: Situated in back of, or in the back part of, or affecting the back or dorsal surface of the body. In lower animals, it refers to the caudal end of the body. [EU]

Practice Guidelines: Directions or principles presenting current or future rules of policy for the health care practitioner to assist him in patient care decisions regarding diagnosis, therapy, or related clinical circumstances. The guidelines may be developed by government agencies at any level, institutions, professional societies, governing boards, or by the convening of expert panels. The guidelines form a basis for the evaluation of all aspects of health care and delivery. [NIH]

Precancerous: A term used to describe a condition that may (or is likely to) become cancer. Also called premalignant. [NIH]

Precursor: Something that precedes. In biological processes, a substance from which another, usually more active or mature substance is formed. In clinical medicine, a sign or symptom that heralds another. [EU]

Predictive factor: A situation or condition that may increase a person's risk of developing a certain disease or disorder. [NIH]

Prednisolone: A glucocorticoid with the general properties of the corticosteroids. It is the drug of choice for all conditions in which routine systemic corticosteroid therapy is indicated, except adrenal deficiency states. [NIH]

Prednisone: A synthetic anti-inflammatory glucocorticoid derived from cortisone. It is biologically inert and converted to prednisolone in the liver. [NIH]

Progesterone: Pregn-4-ene-3,20-dione. The principal progestational hormone of the body, secreted by the corpus luteum, adrenal cortex, and placenta. Its chief function is to prepare the uterus for the reception and development of the fertilized ovum. It acts as an antiovulatory agent when administered on days 5-25 of the menstrual cycle. [NIH]

Progression: Increase in the size of a tumor or spread of cancer in the body. [NIH]

Progressive: Advancing; going forward; going from bad to worse; increasing in scope or severity. [EU]

Projection: A defense mechanism, operating unconsciously, whereby that which is emotionally unacceptable in the self is rejected and attributed (projected) to others. [NIH]

Promoter: A chemical substance that increases the activity of a carcinogenic process. [NIH]

Prophylaxis: An attempt to prevent disease. [NIH]

Prospective study: An epidemiologic study in which a group of individuals (a cohort), all free of a particular disease and varying in their exposure to a possible risk factor, is followed over a specific amount of time to determine the incidence rates of the disease in the exposed and unexposed groups. [NIH]

Protein S: The vitamin K-dependent cofactor of activated protein C. Together with protein C, it inhibits the action of factors VIIIa and Va. A deficiency in protein S can lead to recurrent venous and arterial thrombosis. [NIH]

Proteins: Polymers of amino acids linked by peptide bonds. The specific sequence of amino acids determines the shape and function of the protein. [NIH]

Protozoa: A subkingdom consisting of unicellular organisms that are the simplest in the animal kingdom. Most are free living. They range in size from submicroscopic to macroscopic. Protozoa are divided into seven phyla: Sarcomastigophora, Labyrinthomorpha, Apicomplexa, Microspora, Ascetospora, Myxozoa, and Ciliophora. [NIH]

Protozoal: Having to do with the simplest organisms in the animal kingdom. Protozoa are single-cell organisms, such as ameba, and are different from bacteria, which are not members of the animal kingdom. Some protozoa can be seen without a microscope. [NIH]

Pruritic: Pertaining to or characterized by pruritus. [EU]

Psoriasis: A common genetically determined, chronic, inflammatory skin disease characterized by rounded erythematous, dry, scaling patches. The lesions have a predilection for nails, scalp, genitalia, extensor surfaces, and the lumbosacral region. Accelerated epidermopoiesis is considered to be the fundamental pathologic feature in psoriasis. [NIH]

Ptosis: 1. Prolapse of an organ or part. 2. Drooping of the upper eyelid from paralysis of the third nerve or from sympathetic innervation. [EU]

Public Policy: A course or method of action selected, usually by a government, from among alternatives to guide and determine present and future decisions. [NIH]

Publishing: "The business or profession of the commercial production and issuance of literature" (Webster's 3d). It includes the publisher, publication processes, editing and editors. Production may be by conventional printing methods or by electronic publishing. [NIH]

Pulmonary: Relating to the lungs. [NIH]

Pulse: The rhythmical expansion and contraction of an artery produced by waves of pressure caused by the ejection of blood from the left ventricle of the heart as it contracts. [NIH]

Putrefaction: The process of decomposition of animal and vegetable matter by living organisms. [NIH]

Quality of Life: A generic concept reflecting concern with the modification and enhancement of life attributes, e.g., physical, political, moral and social environment. [NIH]

Radiation: Emission or propagation of electromagnetic energy (waves/rays), or the waves/rays themselves; a stream of electromagnetic particles (electrons, neutrons, protons, alpha particles) or a mixture of these. The most common source is the sun. [NIH]

Radiation therapy: The use of high-energy radiation from x-rays, gamma rays, neutrons, and other sources to kill cancer cells and shrink tumors. Radiation may come from a machine outside the body (external-beam radiation therapy), or it may come from radioactive material placed in the body in the area near cancer cells (internal radiation therapy, implant radiation, or brachytherapy). Systemic radiation therapy uses a radioactive substance, such as a radiolabeled monoclonal antibody, that circulates throughout the body. Also called radiotherapy. [NIH]

Radicular: Having the character of or relating to a radicle or root. [NIH]

Radiculopathy: Disease involving a spinal nerve root (see spinal nerve roots) which may result from compression related to intervertebral disk displacement; spinal cord injuries; spinal diseases; and other conditions. Clinical manifestations include radicular pain, weakness, and sensory loss referable to structures innervated by the involved nerve root. [NIH]

Radiological: Pertaining to radiodiagnostic and radiotherapeutic procedures, and interventional radiology or other planning and guiding medical radiology. [NIH]

Randomized: Describes an experiment or clinical trial in which animal or human subjects are assigned by chance to separate groups that compare different treatments. [NIH]

Receptor: A molecule inside or on the surface of a cell that binds to a specific substance and causes a specific physiologic effect in the cell. [NIH]

Rectum: The last 8 to 10 inches of the large intestine. [NIH]

Recurrence: The return of a sign, symptom, or disease after a remission. [NIH]

Reductase: Enzyme converting testosterone to dihydrotestosterone. [NIH]

Refer: To send or direct for treatment, aid, information, de decision. [NIH]

Refraction: A test to determine the best eyeglasses or contact lenses to correct a refractive error (myopia, hyperopia, or astigmatism). [NIH]

Regeneration: The natural renewal of a structure, as of a lost tissue or part. [EU]

Reliability: Used technically, in a statistical sense, of consistency of a test with itself, i. e. the extent to which we can assume that it will yield the same result if repeated a second time. [NIH]

Remission: A decrease in or disappearance of signs and symptoms of cancer. In partial remission, some, but not all, signs and symptoms of cancer have disappeared. In complete remission, all signs and symptoms of cancer have disappeared, although there still may be cancer in the body. [NIH]

Renal failure: Progressive renal insufficiency and uremia, due to irreversible and progressive renal glomerular tubular or interstitial disease. [NIH]

Retina: The ten-layered nervous tissue membrane of the eye. It is continuous with the optic nerve and receives images of external objects and transmits visual impulses to the brain. Its outer surface is in contact with the choroid and the inner surface with the vitreous body. The outer-most layer is pigmented, whereas the inner nine layers are transparent. [NIH]

Retinal: 1. Pertaining to the retina. 2. The aldehyde of retinol, derived by the oxidative enzymatic splitting of absorbed dietary carotene, and having vitamin A activity. In the retina, retinal combines with opsins to form visual pigments. One isomer, 11-cis retinal combines with opsin in the rods (scotopsin) to form rhodopsin, or visual purple. Another, all-trans retinal (trans-r.); visual yellow; xanthopsin) results from the bleaching of rhodopsin by light, in which the 11-cis form is converted to the all-trans form. Retinal also combines with opsins in the cones (photopsins) to form the three pigments responsible for colour vision. Called also retinal, and retinene1. [EU]

Retinal Artery: Central retinal artery and its branches. It arises from the ophthalmic artery, pierces the optic nerve and runs through its center, enters the eye through the porus opticus and branches to supply the retina. [NIH]

Retinal Artery Occlusion: Occlusion or closure of the central retinal artery causing sudden, usually nearly complete, loss of vision in one eye. Occlusion of the branch retinal artery causes sudden visual loss in only a portion of the visual field. [NIH]

Retinal Ganglion Cells: Cells of the innermost nuclear layer of the retina, the ganglion cell layer, which project axons through the optic nerve to the brain. They are quite variable in size and in the shapes of their dendritic arbors, which are generally confined to the inner plexiform layer. [NIH]

Retinol: Vitamin A. It is essential for proper vision and healthy skin and mucous membranes. Retinol is being studied for cancer prevention; it belongs to the family of drugs called retinoids. [NIH]

Rheumatism: A group of disorders marked by inflammation or pain in the connective tissue structures of the body. These structures include bone, cartilage, and fat. [NIH]

Rheumatoid: Resembling rheumatism. [EU]

Rheumatoid arthritis: A form of arthritis, the cause of which is unknown, although infection, hypersensitivity, hormone imbalance and psychologic stress have been suggested as possible causes. [NIH]

Rheumatology: A subspecialty of internal medicine concerned with the study of inflammatory or degenerative processes and metabolic derangement of connective tissue structures which pertain to a variety of musculoskeletal disorders, such as arthritis. [NIH]

Rhodopsin: A photoreceptor protein found in retinal rods. It is a complex formed by the binding of retinal, the oxidized form of retinol, to the protein opsin and undergoes a series of complex reactions in response to visible light resulting in the transmission of nerve impulses to the brain. [NIH]

Risk factor: A habit, trait, condition, or genetic alteration that increases a person's chance of developing a disease. [NIH]

Rods: One type of specialized light-sensitive cells (photoreceptors) in the retina that provide side vision and the ability to see objects in dim light (night vision). [NIH]

Salivary: The duct that convey saliva to the mouth. [NIH]

Salivary glands: Glands in the mouth that produce saliva. [NIH]

Saponins: Sapogenin glycosides. A type of glycoside widely distributed in plants. Each consists of a sapogenin as the aglycon moiety, and a sugar. The sapogenin may be a steroid or a triterpene and the sugar may be glucose, galactose, a pentose, or a methylpentose. Sapogenins are poisonous towards the lower forms of life and are powerful hemolytics when injected into the blood stream able to dissolve red blood cells at even extreme dilutions. [NIH]

Scleroderma: A chronic disorder marked by hardening and thickening of the skin. Scleroderma can be localized or it can affect the entire body (systemic). [NIH]

Screening: Checking for disease when there are no symptoms. [NIH]

Secretion: 1. The process of elaborating a specific product as a result of the activity of a gland; this activity may range from separating a specific substance of the blood to the elaboration of a new chemical substance. 2. Any substance produced by secretion. [EU]

Sediment: A precipitate, especially one that is formed spontaneously. [EU]

Sedimentation: The act of causing the deposit of sediment, especially by the use of a centrifugal machine. [EU]

Senile: Relating or belonging to old age; characteristic of old age; resulting from infirmity of old age. [NIH]

Sensory loss: A disease of the nerves whereby the myelin or insulating sheath of myelin on the nerves does not stay intact and the messages from the brain to the muscles through the nerves are not carried properly. [NIH]

Sequencing: The determination of the order of nucleotides in a DNA or RNA chain. [NIH]

Serum: The clear liquid part of the blood that remains after blood cells and clotting proteins have been removed. [NIH]

Shock: The general bodily disturbance following a severe injury; an emotional or moral upset occasioned by some disturbing or unexpected experience; disruption of the circulation, which can upset all body functions: sometimes referred to as circulatory shock. [NIH]

Sialorrhea: Increased salivary flow. [NIH]

Sicca: Failure of lacrimal secretion, keratoconjunctivitis sicca, failure of secretion of the salivary glands and mucous glands of the upper respiratory tract and polyarthritis. [NIH]

Side effect: A consequence other than the one(s) for which an agent or measure is used, as the adverse effects produced by a drug, especially on a tissue or organ system other than the one sought to be benefited by its administration. [EU]

Sigmoid: 1. Shaped like the letter S or the letter C. 2. The sigmoid colon. [EU]

Sigmoid Colon: The lower part of the colon that empties into the rectum. [NIH]

Signs and Symptoms: Clinical manifestations that can be either objective when observed by a physician, or subjective when perceived by the patient. [NIH]

Skeleton: The framework that supports the soft tissues of vertebrate animals and protects many of their internal organs. The skeletons of vertebrates are made of bone and/or cartilage. [NIH]

Skull: The skeleton of the head including the bones of the face and the bones enclosing the brain. [NIH]

Skull Neoplasms: Neoplasms of the bony part of the skull. [NIH]

Small intestine: The part of the digestive tract that is located between the stomach and the large intestine. [NIH]

Social Environment: The aggregate of social and cultural institutions, forms, patterns, and processes that influence the life of an individual or community. [NIH]

Specialist: In medicine, one who concentrates on 1 special branch of medical science. [NIH]

Species: A taxonomic category subordinate to a genus (or subgenus) and superior to a subspecies or variety, composed of individuals possessing common characters distinguishing them from other categories of individuals of the same taxonomic level. In taxonomic nomenclature, species are designated by the genus name followed by a Latin or Latinized adjective or noun. [EU]

Spectrum: A charted band of wavelengths of electromagnetic vibrations obtained by refraction and diffraction. By extension, a measurable range of activity, such as the range of bacteria affected by an antibiotic (antibacterial s.) or the complete range of manifestations of a disease. [EU]

Spinal cord: The main trunk or bundle of nerves running down the spine through holes in the spinal bone (the vertebrae) from the brain to the level of the lower back. [NIH]

Spinal Nerve Roots: The paired bundles of nerve fibers entering and leaving the spinal cord at each segment. The dorsal and ventral nerve roots join to form the mixed segmental spinal nerves. The dorsal roots are generally afferent, formed by the central projections of the spinal (dorsal root) ganglia sensory cells, and the ventral roots efferent, comprising the axons of spinal motor and autonomic preganglionic neurons. There are, however, some exceptions to this afferent/efferent rule. [NIH]

Spleen: An organ that is part of the lymphatic system. The spleen produces lymphocytes, filters the blood, stores blood cells, and destroys old blood cells. It is located on the left side of the abdomen near the stomach. [NIH]

Squamous: Scaly, or platelike. [EU]

Squamous cell carcinoma: Cancer that begins in squamous cells, which are thin, flat cells resembling fish scales. Squamous cells are found in the tissue that forms the surface of the skin, the lining of the hollow organs of the body, and the passages of the respiratory and digestive tracts. Also called epidermoid carcinoma. [NIH]

Squamous cell carcinoma: Cancer that begins in squamous cells, which are thin, flat cells resembling fish scales. Squamous cells are found in the tissue that forms the surface of the skin, the lining of the hollow organs of the body, and the passages of the respiratory and digestive tracts. Also called epidermoid carcinoma. [NIH]

Squamous cells: Flat cells that look like fish scales under a microscope. These cells cover internal and external surfaces of the body. [NIH]

Stabilization: The creation of a stable state. [EU]

Stenosis: Narrowing or stricture of a duct or canal. [EU]

Steroid: A group name for lipids that contain a hydrogenated cyclopentanoperhydrophenanthrene ring system. Some of the substances included in this group are progesterone, adrenocortical hormones, the gonadal hormones, cardiac aglycones, bile acids, sterols (such as cholesterol), toad poisons, saponins, and some of the carcinogenic hydrocarbons. [EU]

Steroid therapy: Treatment with corticosteroid drugs to reduce swelling, pain, and other symptoms of inflammation. [NIH]

Stimulus: That which can elicit or evoke action (response) in a muscle, nerve, gland or other excitable issue, or cause an augmenting action upon any function or metabolic process. [NIH]

Stomach: An organ of digestion situated in the left upper quadrant of the abdomen between the termination of the esophagus and the beginning of the duodenum. [NIH]

Stomatitis: Inflammation of the oral mucosa, due to local or systemic factors which may involve the buccal and labial mucosa, palate, tongue, floor of the mouth, and the gingivae. [EU]

Strand: DNA normally exists in the bacterial nucleus in a helix, in which two strands are coiled together. [NIH]

Stress: Forcibly exerted influence; pressure. Any condition or situation that causes strain or tension. Stress may be either physical or psychologic, or both. [NIH]

Stricture: The abnormal narrowing of a body opening. Also called stenosis. [NIH]

Stroke: Sudden loss of function of part of the brain because of loss of blood flow. Stroke may be caused by a clot (thrombosis) or rupture (hemorrhage) of a blood vessel to the brain. [NIH]

Subacute: Somewhat acute; between acute and chronic. [EU]

Subarachnoid: Situated or occurring between the arachnoid and the pia mater. [EU]

Subclavian: The direct continuation of the axillary vein at the lateral border of the first rib. It passes medially to join the internal jugular vein and form the brachiocephalic vein on each side. [NIH]

Subclavian Artery: Artery arising from the brachiocephalic trunk on the right side and from the arch of the aorta on the left side. It distributes to the neck, thoracic wall, spinal cord, brain, meninges, and upper limb. [NIH]

Subclinical: Without clinical manifestations; said of the early stage(s) of an infection or other disease or abnormality before symptoms and signs become apparent or detectable by clinical examination or laboratory tests, or of a very mild form of an infection or other disease or abnormality. [EU]

Subcutaneous: Beneath the skin. [NIH]

Submucous: Occurring beneath the mucosa or a mucous membrane. [NIH]

Suppression: A conscious exclusion of disapproved desire contrary with repression, in which the process of exclusion is not conscious. [NIH]

Syncytium: A living nucleated tissue without apparent cellular structure; a tissue composed of a mass of nucleated protoplasm without cell boundaries. [NIH]

Systemic: Affecting the entire body. [NIH]

Systemic disease: Disease that affects the whole body. [NIH]

Temporal: One of the two irregular bones forming part of the lateral surfaces and base of the skull, and containing the organs of hearing. [NIH]

Temporal Arteries: Arteries arising from the external carotid or the maxillary artery and distributing to the temporal region. [NIH]

Tendon: A discrete band of connective tissue mainly composed of parallel bundles of collagenous fibers by which muscles are attached, or two muscles bellies joined. [NIH]

Tetanus: A disease caused by tetanospasmin, a powerful protein toxin produced by Clostridium tetani. Tetanus usually occurs after an acute injury, such as a puncture wound or laceration. Generalized tetanus, the most common form, is characterized by tetanic muscular contractions and hyperreflexia. Localized tetanus presents itself as a mild condition with manifestations restricted to muscles near the wound. It may progress to the generalized form. [NIH]

Thermal: Pertaining to or characterized by heat. [EU]

Thigh: A leg; in anatomy, any elongated process or part of a structure more or less comparable to a leg. [NIH]

Thoracic: Having to do with the chest. [NIH]

Thorax: A part of the trunk between the neck and the abdomen; the chest. [NIH]

Thrombocytosis: Increased numbers of platelets in the peripheral blood. [EU]

Thrombosis: The formation or presence of a blood clot inside a blood vessel. [NIH]

Thrombus: An aggregation of blood factors, primarily platelets and fibrin with entrapment of cellular elements, frequently causing vascular obstruction at the point of its formation. Some authorities thus differentiate thrombus formation from simple coagulation or clot formation. [EU]

Tinnitus: Sounds that are perceived in the absence of any external noise source which may take the form of buzzing, ringing, clicking, pulsations, and other noises. Objective tinnitus refers to noises generated from within the ear or adjacent structures that can be heard by other individuals. The term subjective tinnitus is used when the sound is audible only to the affected individual. Tinnitus may occur as a manifestation of cochlear diseases;

vestibulocochlear nerve diseases; intracranial hypertension; craniocerebral trauma; and other conditions. [NIH]

Tissue: A group or layer of cells that are alike in type and work together to perform a specific function. [NIH]

Tolerance: 1. The ability to endure unusually large doses of a drug or toxin. 2. Acquired drug tolerance; a decreasing response to repeated constant doses of a drug or the need for increasing doses to maintain a constant response. [EU]

Tomography: Imaging methods that result in sharp images of objects located on a chosen plane and blurred images located above or below the plane. [NIH]

Torsion: A twisting or rotation of a bodily part or member on its axis. [NIH]

Toxic: Having to do with poison or something harmful to the body. Toxic substances usually cause unwanted side effects. [NIH]

Toxicology: The science concerned with the detection, chemical composition, and pharmacologic action of toxic substances or poisons and the treatment and prevention of toxic manifestations. [NIH]

Toxin: A poison; frequently used to refer specifically to a protein produced by some higher plants, certain animals, and pathogenic bacteria, which is highly toxic for other living organisms. Such substances are differentiated from the simple chemical poisons and the vegetable alkaloids by their high molecular weight and antigenicity. [EU]

Transfection: The uptake of naked or purified DNA into cells, usually eukaryotic. It is analogous to bacterial transformation. [NIH]

Trauma: Any injury, wound, or shock, must frequently physical or structural shock, producing a disturbance. [NIH]

Trismus: Spasmodic contraction of the masseter muscle resulting in forceful jaw closure. This may be seen with a variety of diseases, including tetanus, as a complication of radiation therapy, trauma, or in association with neoplastic conditions. [NIH]

Tuberculosis: Any of the infectious diseases of man and other animals caused by species of Mycobacterium. [NIH]

Tumor Necrosis Factor: Serum glycoprotein produced by activated macrophages and other mammalian mononuclear leukocytes which has necrotizing activity against tumor cell lines and increases ability to reject tumor transplants. It mimics the action of endotoxin but differs from it. It has a molecular weight of less than 70,000 kDa. [NIH]

Tumour: 1. Swelling, one of the cardinal signs of inflammations; morbid enlargement. 2. A new growth of tissue in which the multiplication of cells is uncontrolled and progressive; called also neoplasm. [EU]

Tunica: A rather vague term to denote the lining coat of hollow organs, tubes, or cavities. [NIH]

Ulcer: A localized necrotic lesion of the skin or a mucous surface. [NIH]

Ultrasonography: The visualization of deep structures of the body by recording the reflections of echoes of pulses of ultrasonic waves directed into the tissues. Use of ultrasound for imaging or diagnostic purposes employs frequencies ranging from 1.6 to 10 megahertz. [NIH]

Uremia: The illness associated with the buildup of urea in the blood because the kidneys are not working effectively. Symptoms include nausea, vomiting, loss of appetite, weakness, and mental confusion. [NIH]

Urine: Fluid containing water and waste products. Urine is made by the kidneys, stored in the bladder, and leaves the body through the urethra. [NIH]

Urticaria: A vascular reaction of the skin characterized by erythema and wheal formation due to localized increase of vascular permeability. The causative mechanism may be allergy, infection, or stress. [NIH]

Uterus: The small, hollow, pear-shaped organ in a woman's pelvis. This is the organ in which a fetus develops. Also called the womb. [NIH]

Vaccination: Administration of vaccines to stimulate the host's immune response. This includes any preparation intended for active immunological prophylaxis. [NIH]

Vaccines: Suspensions of killed or attenuated microorganisms (bacteria, viruses, fungi, protozoa, or rickettsiae), antigenic proteins derived from them, or synthetic constructs, administered for the prevention, amelioration, or treatment of infectious and other diseases. [NIH]

Varicella: Chicken pox. [EU]

Vasa Vasorum: Nutrient blood vessels which supply the walls of large arteries or veins. [NIH]

Vascular: Pertaining to blood vessels or indicative of a copious blood supply. [EU]

Vasculitis: Inflammation of a blood vessel. [NIH]

Vasodilators: Any nerve or agent which induces dilatation of the blood vessels. [NIH]

Vector: Plasmid or other self-replicating DNA molecule that transfers DNA between cells in nature or in recombinant DNA technology. [NIH]

Vein: Vessel-carrying blood from various parts of the body to the heart. [NIH]

Venous: Of or pertaining to the veins. [EU]

Ventral: 1. Pertaining to the belly or to any venter. 2. Denoting a position more toward the belly surface than some other object of reference; same as anterior in human anatomy. [EU]

Ventricle: One of the two pumping chambers of the heart. The right ventricle receives oxygen-poor blood from the right atrium and pumps it to the lungs through the pulmonary artery. The left ventricle receives oxygen-rich blood from the left atrium and pumps it to the body through the aorta. [NIH]

Venules: The minute vessels that collect blood from the capillary plexuses and join together to form veins. [NIH]

Vertebrae: A bony unit of the segmented spinal column. [NIH]

Vertebral: Of or pertaining to a vertebra. [EU]

Vertebral Artery: The first branch of the subclavian artery with distribution to muscles of the neck, vertebrae, spinal cord, cerebellum and interior of the cerebrum. [NIH]

Vertigo: An illusion of movement; a sensation as if the external world were revolving around the patient (objective vertigo) or as if he himself were revolving in space (subjective vertigo). The term is sometimes erroneously used to mean any form of dizziness. [EU]

Vesicular: 1. Composed of or relating to small, saclike bodies. 2. Pertaining to or made up of vesicles on the skin. [EU]

Veterinary Medicine: The medical science concerned with the prevention, diagnosis, and treatment of diseases in animals. [NIH]

Viral: Pertaining to, caused by, or of the nature of virus. [EU]

Virus: Submicroscopic organism that causes infectious disease. In cancer therapy, some viruses may be made into vaccines that help the body build an immune response to, and kill, tumor cells. [NIH]

Visual field: The entire area that can be seen when the eye is forward, including peripheral vision. [NIH]

Vitro: Descriptive of an event or enzyme reaction under experimental investigation occurring outside a living organism. Parts of an organism or microorganism are used together with artificial substrates and/or conditions. [NIH]

War: Hostile conflict between organized groups of people. [NIH]

White blood cell: A type of cell in the immune system that helps the body fight infection and disease. White blood cells include lymphocytes, granulocytes, macrophages, and others. [NIH]

Womb: A hollow, thick-walled, muscular organ in which the impregnated ovum is developed into a child. [NIH]

Wound Healing: Restoration of integrity to traumatized tissue. [NIH]

Xenograft: The cells of one species transplanted to another species. [NIH]

Xerostomia: Decreased salivary flow. [NIH]

Zoster: A virus infection of the Gasserian ganglion and its nerve branches, characterized by discrete areas of vesiculation of the epithelium of the forehead, the nose, the eyelids, and the cornea together with subepithelial infiltration. [NIH]

INDEX

p.102 Oculomotor nerve

p.16 disparate results in studies of methotrexate

p.16 distinct vascular lesions

p.20 facial edema

p.23 GCA clues to early diagnosis

24 GCA oculomotor nerve palsy

p.25 GCA diagnosis

p.25 Heeding clues

Printed in the United States
112731LV00004B/6/A